Dear Tom,

Thank you for ___
when my neck was at its worst.
You literally saved my neck,

PATIENTLY WAITING FOR...

and I think of you frequently.
I hope you'll like this book
I know you'll like the book's
purpose.

Again thanks

Jeff

PATIENTLY WAITING FOR...

JEFF NISKER

IGUANA

Copyright © 2015 Jeff Nisker
Published by Iguana Books
720 Bathurst Street, Suite 303
Toronto, Ontario, Canada
M5V 2R4

All rights reserved. No part of this publication may be reproduced, stored in a retrieval system or transmitted, in any form or by any means, electronic, mechanical, recording or otherwise (except brief passages for purposes of review) without the prior permission of the author or a licence from The Canadian Copyright Licensing Agency (Access Copyright). For an Access Copyright licence, visit www.accesscopyright.ca or call toll free to 1-800-893-5777.

Publisher: Greg Ioannou
Editor: Mariko Obokata
Front cover design and illustration: Angela Vaculik
Book layout design: Caitlin Stewart

Library and Archives Canada Cataloguing in Publication

Nisker, Jeffrey A., author
    Patiently waiting for ... / J. Nisker.

Issued in print and electronic formats.
ISBN 978-1-77180-136-2 (paperback).--ISBN 978-1-77180-137-9 (epub).--ISBN 978-1-77180-138-6 (kindle)

    I. Title.

PS8627.I85P38 2015   C813'.6   C2015-906180-6
                                                      C2015-906181-4

This is an original print edition of *Patiently Waiting For* ...

To Catherine Frazee and the woman I call Ruth.

Let your life speak

Traditional Quaker saying

Table of Contents

Introduction i
Preface vii
Chapter 1   0120 h, May 1, 2000 1
Chapter 2   November 15, 1997 3
Chapter 3   November 15, 1997 10
Chapter 4   February 6, 1998 13
Chapter 5   November 15, 1997 18
Chapter 6   February 7, 1998 23
Chapter 7   February 8, 1998 26
Chapter 8   May 6, 2000 37
Chapter 9   February 9, 1998 39
Chapter 10   February 9, 1998 42
Chapter 11   May 6, 2000 45
Chapter 12   November 16, 1997 46
Chapter 13   January 30, 1999 48
Chapter 14   April 27, 1998 50
Chapter 15   April 27, 1998 57
Chapter 16   May 6, 2000 66
Chapter 17   September 28, 1998 67
Chapter 18   September 28, 1998 69
Chapter 19   September 28, 1998 70
Chapter 20   May 6, 2000 73
Chapter 21   September 28, 1998 74
Chapter 22   September 28, 1998 79
Chapter 23   September 28, 1998 81

Chapter 24	May 6, 2000	84
Chapter 25	October 1, 1998	85
Chapter 26	October 2, 1998	89
Chapter 27	May 6, 2000	92
Chapter 28	November 25, 1999	94
Chapter 29	October 2, 1998	99
Chapter 30	December 10, 1999	101
Chapter 31	October 2, 1998	106
Chapter 32	February 5, 2000	108
Chapter 33	February 17, 2000	110
Chapter 34	May 6, 2000	112
Chapter 35	February 22, 2000	113
Chapter 36	April 27, 2000	115
Chapter 37	1330 h, April 30, 2000	117
Chapter 38	May 6, 2000	121
Chapter 39	2210 h, April 30, 2000	122
Chapter 40	0120 h, May 1, 2000	124
Chapter 41	May 6, 2000	128
Epilogue	Spring 2005	130
Afterword		139
Acknowledgements		145
Popular References		147
Scholarly References		151
Further Readings		153
About the Author		159

Introduction

Jackie Leach Scully

"The day I get hooked up to my computer will be the first day of my beautiful new life."

That quote, from the narrative voiced by Ruth in *Patiently Waiting For…*, encapsulates the central claim, problem, and injustice compellingly described in this book. It guides us toward one of the important points that Jeff Nisker makes in his complex and nuanced fictional account "based on true occurrences" of the relationship (of sorts) between a quadriplegic woman he calls Ruth and a doctor. A fiction like Jeff Nisker's doesn't make arguments in the standard academic way. Instead, he uses narrative as a starting point for thought; alongside telling a story, this book forces its readers to think harder about what they may have taken for granted about their own and other people's attitudes to disability, quality of life, social responsibility, power, euthanasia, and death.

Writing an introduction to a piece like this book is not easy. It should whet the reader's appetite for carrying on with it, but not give away so much of the plot that all narrative tension is destroyed. It should, ideally, indicate why reading the book will be enjoyable or useful, or both, but not do so by pre-empting what the author will go on to say in a more extended (and probably more entertaining) fashion. Here are some of what I identify as the significant themes that I'm sure I will return to think about in the future; they "spoke to my condition," as the

Quakers say. Other readers are likely to see different highlights, reflecting their own perspectives and priorities.

The narrative describes the doctor's growing sensitivity to the factors that shape the realities of life for people with disabilities. What matters as much or more than just the biology of difference and impairment, which is of course the natural focus of biomedical concern, are our individual and societal responses to disability. Ruth experiences the commonplace physical and social marginalization and the routine disrespect that too many people with disabilities have no choice but to endure, whether through the exposure of intimate parts of her body without her knowledge or consent, the neglect of her clearly expressed needs and desires, or the alacrity with which her professional carers make judgements about her quality of life.

It was the work of disability activists, and of the theorists who developed increasingly sophisticated accounts of what constitutes *disability* in the first place, that now makes it possible to think of *disability* as a complex interaction between one's biology (the body's physical or physiological anomaly) and one's environment. At best, this interaction encourages the flourishing of a level of creativity that can effectively re-imagine how the world could be if the norms of disability were accepted as more universally applicable. At worst, it results in people with disabilities facing insurmountable material, economic, social, imaginative, and other barriers to their possibilities of being fully functional, integrated, creative members of their societies.

Set in Canada in the late 1990s, healthcare and disability support are in crisis "because of the slash of health funding since the last election to fulfill the campaign promise of personal income tax breaks." The political details are specific to the time and place of the narrative, but the overall message is more widely relevant. In today's complex and managed societies, it's provision of money and resources that determines overall "quality of life," more than the chances of biology; and the directions in which money and resources flow are the end result of political choices that in turn reflect deeply engrained social and cultural attitudes. The infections that propel Ruth onto the emergency ward are the indirect result of staffing cuts in the group home, because they mean she doesn't get turned frequently enough to prevent bedsores developing.

The focal point of the drama is Ruth's patient wait for an intervention that will enable her to communicate beyond the four walls of her room. This is a necessity of life, not a luxury, for Ruth. The delay is not because of a malevolent desire to deprive her, but because of a lack of resources to make it happen, and ultimately the lack of will to redirect resources to support the lives of people with disabilities. As I write this introduction more than 15 years after the events of the story, not much has changed for the better. Alongside a generally improved awareness of disability and of disability rights, the post-2008 global economic downturn has created a climate in which people with disabilities are still among the last to experience the resources that would enable them to flourish as equal citizens, and the first to have those resources withdrawn.

One aspect of the doctor–patient relationship that this book highlights is the limits to the knowledge that one person can have about another — whether that is factual knowledge about someone's life situation, their medical condition and prognosis, or, as in this story, a more intangible subjective grasp of their experiential world: what it is like to be *them*. The notion of epistemic humility — that is, being deliberately modest about the claims you can make in terms of grasping the realities of someone else's life — is becoming familiar to epistemological theory; it's much more rarely introduced in the biomedical context. In reality, doctors tend not to know much about their patients beyond the clinical details. Often, patients know just as little about their doctors, although Ruth, aided by her long immersion in the medical world and her acute eye, is an exception. (And it might be said that such ignorance, on the part of patients, matters less to clinical outcomes anyway.)

This limit of knowledge first shows up here when Jeff Nisker notes that although the text is "built on true occurrences," it is neither an accurate factual account nor completely fictional, because to offer it as either would be to "presume more insight into [Ruth's] lived experience than I could possibly possess." The moral and political arrogance of such an assumption, as Nisker recognizes, is increasingly recognized as a major point of tension within disability studies, notably in memoirs that chronicle experiences of disability and illness. In many cases (especially when the story concerns intellectual impairment, severe barriers to communication, or terminal illness), the account *has* to be written by a third party — a family member, less often a clinician — and here the author can be suspected of claiming the right to *speak for* the disabled or ill person, raising all sorts of issues of knowledge, power and voice.

Jeff Nisker's book alternates between the perspective of the doctor and that of Ruth, but he carefully emphasizes that he is not claiming to voice the truth of either; his aim is to produce a compelling narrative. The book quite deliberately raises uncomfortable questions about persons with disabilities, nondisabled people, power, and exploitation. (Indeed, Nisker alludes to this discussion when he says, "Ruth was not permitted her voice, so she was forced to use mine." Ruth did in fact ask Jeff the author to tell her story, and even to use her real name, although he chose not to do so.) The uncomfortable questions are there from the outset, starting with the doctor's desire to be Ruth's friend rather than her physician. He steps aside from the physician role in order to dissolve the doctor–patient bond and remove the power differential inherent within it. But he remains a doctor, even if not *her* doctor; Ruth remains a patient, even if they become, to some extent, friends; and that power differential cannot be completely dismantled.

The doctor asks, "Is there anything you need, Ruth?" And at this point he genuinely believes that, as a doctor and (more saliently) an able-bodied person, he has the power to make things happen for her; all she has to do is ask. This common but problematic delusion of omnipotence among the nondisabled is the mirror image of the deeply held, toxic conviction that people with disabilities are inescapably helpless and vulnerable. In fact, as it turns out, the one thing that Ruth explicitly asks the doctor to help her with is something that he *can't* make happen for her. This is the "failure" that resurfaces throughout the book, described from the outset as the story of "how I let her down." The reader, however, can take a wider perspective, and will realize that the doctor here is being unnecessarily hard on himself. Although there may have been some personal failures on his part, a degree of paternalism and patronization, the fact that he can't provide what she needs so desperately is as much the responsibility of the existing health and support systems as any failing of his.

Authors writing on disability today raise profound questions about awareness, inclusion, and the fundamental difficulties we seem to have with difference and impairment. But despite this broadening of scope, there is still little engagement with what might be described as the spiritual dimension of responses to difference and discrimination. Here, Jeff Nisker's account takes a distinctive direction. Toward the end of this story, Ruth has become part of her local Quaker meeting, and the narrative returns several times to the doctor's experiences at a memorial Quaker meeting. As in many Quaker meetings, this memorial service is held in an "unprogrammed" fashion. There is no minister and no liturgy, and verbal contributions — which are often informal and anecdotal — are made by those present if they are led to do so as they "wait on God."

Quakerism is a distinctive religious path for a number of reasons, but perhaps most relevant to Ruth's story is its longstanding "testimony to equality." Right from its origins in the seventeenth century, an explicit commitment to the equality of all people has been a cornerstone of Quaker belief and practice; it's an ideal that hasn't always been lived up to, but it has endured and its reach expanded. In principle then, the Quaker commitment to equality today includes the taken-for-granted inclusion of people with disabilities within the Quaker and wider human community, and in practice, that means significant time and effort now being directed toward changing environments and attitudes to make this possible.

By tying Quakerism to Ruth's story, Nisker ensures that readers make an important connection not with a particular faith group, but between the way in which a society treats people with disabilities and that society's foundational beliefs about who belongs in the community, how far someone can differ from the community norm before they stop belonging, and how far we are willing to go to ensure everyone is treated with equality.

Patiently Waiting For ... contains a rich variety of starting points for fresh thinking about difference and our responses to it in the healthcare setting. Above all, Jeff Nisker embeds these catalysts within a *story*, sharing the conviction of many bioethicists today that narrative provides an essential complement to more abstract theoretical reasoning. In Ruth's story, we are confronted with the full complexity and untidiness of real-life ethical tensions, where situations can be morally troubling without fitting comfortably into the structure of an "ethical dilemma." Ruth's "doctor-friend" is not faced with an ethical either/or, but he *is* called upon to scrutinize his moral and professional obligations, relationships, and capacities, and to live with the inadequacy of the response he as an individual is able to make. Inadequate but perhaps, in the circumstances, the best that he can do.

Preface

Patiently Waiting For ... is a work of fiction built on true occurrences in the life of a woman who asked me to write her story, and true occurrences in my sound-bite relationship with her. She asked me to write her story so that others will have a different story: a story free of the denial of access so prominent in her story, a story free of the consequences that accompany such denial. She instructed me to use her real name but I have not, so as not to conflate fiction with fact or presume more insight into her lived experience than I could possibly possess. As she asked me to write her story, I have written *Patiently Waiting For* ... with as much of her permission as possible, considering she did not live to read even the first words I wrote about her, the words I was asked to speak at her memorial service. *Patiently Waiting For* ... is my much put-off attempt to fulfill my promise to this woman. I have tried to write the story I think she wanted me to write.

Patiently Waiting For ... is also built on true occurrences in my friendship with Catherine Frazee, a disabilities scholar, activist, and university professor. Catherine has read *Patiently Waiting For* ... and given me permission to use her name and to include my first experience of her in this book. Catherine's insight inspired, her kindness encouraged, and her wisdom is woven throughout the book. I hope I have written a book worthy of her friendship. *Patiently Waiting For* ... is dedicated to these two wonderful women.

When this book goes to press, it will have been over fifteen years since the woman represented as the central character asked me to write her story. Over those years, I started writing her story many times, but was always diverted by my other "responsibilities." Perhaps I had conveniently allowed myself to be diverted because I knew writing her story would insist I explore not only how our health and social support systems let her down but how I let her down. I would have to explore a part of me that I preferred remain submerged, a part of me that was as bad as our country's health and social policy in confining her in a prison of possibility denied.

I was asked if I might say a few words at her memorial service. Soon after, based on those words, I published an article in the *Canadian Medical Association Journal* as my attempt to bring to the attention of those responsible for health and social policy the inadequacies in the health promotion, accommodation, and social support she had received. However, the 1000-word limit assaulted any ability to convey the person she was, and trying to know her is essential to appreciate the injustices of the lack of accommodation and denial of health promotion promulgated upon her. She must have understood the importance of personal story to humane policy development or she would not have asked me to write her personal story.

Since her death, the inequality of access to assistive technologies she experienced has greatly intensified, as each new technology, by increasing the possibilities, has widened the divide between those who have the financial means to pay for these technologies and those who do not. These inequalities in access are indeed increasingly inflicted by one of the world's wealthiest countries and its supposedly wonderful health and social support systems on its socioeconomically disadvantaged citizens, among whom disabled citizens are highly overrepresented. The fact that this discrimination in access to these technologies occurs in a country with a Charter of Rights and Freedoms forged in fairness and anti-discrimination, a country that signed the United Nations Convention on the Rights of Persons with Disabilities, whose Articles specifically address the discrimination found in *Patiently Waiting For* ..., suggests Canada and likely many other so-called "developed" countries have become places where the imperative to personal wealth has displaced communal caring and social justice.

Portions of *Patiently Waiting For* ... have appeared in play form in *From Calcedonies to Orchids: Plays Promoting Humanity in Health Policy* (Iguana Books) and *Health Humanities Reader* (Rutgers University Press); and in essay form in the *Canadian Medical Association Journal* (January 2001). See Further Readings for details on these publications.

Chapter 1

0120 h, May 1, 2000

I quietly open the front door to my home. My feet magnetically move to my answering machine. No red light flashing, but there is a note beside it from my youngest: "Hospital has been looking for you Dad going to bed."
    I'm not on call. Must be some mistake.
    I phone the Hospital and page the resident on call. A sleepy voice answers, "Hello."
    "I'm sorry to wake you up, but are you looking for me?"
    "No. You're not covering tonight are you?"
    "No. Again I'm sorry for waking you."
    The Hospital must have called me by mistake. Some confusion now rectified.
    I walk to my bedroom, throw my jacket on the chair, kick off my shoes, and fall back on the bed, eyes are already shut.
    I wake to the phone ringing.
    "Yes."
    "Ruth's in trouble," a woman's voice whispers urgently. "Please come to the hospital right away."
    I hear a dial tone. I see that it's 3:00 a.m.
    I quickly put on my jacket and shoes, and speed to the Hospital. I park illegally at the ER doors and run in. The woman at ER reception tells me Ruth is not there, and hasn't been since she came on at seven. Good. Ruth must have been admitted. I ask the receptionist which room Ruth is in. Her computer is taking too long. I run up the stairs and down the hall to Intensive Care.

2 Patiently Waiting For ...

The nurse at the desk seems to be expecting me. She appears frightened. She doesn't say anything. Instead, her eyes move from mine to look down at the index finger of her right hand. It is pointing to a draped-off area at the Unit's far end, about fifty metres away. I turn my head and see incandescent curtains projecting ominous shadows. I turn my body to dash there, but the nurse grips my right wrist hard, while gently whispering in a soothing but frightened voice, "Why don't you stay here with me until they're finished?"

Chapter 2

November 15, 1997

Calcedonies wait. They patiently wait.... Calcedonies are rocks. Crusty-surfaced, irregular-shaped rocks. Rocks that open up to amethyst or onyx or agate or chrysoprase. Rocks that become amulets or jewellery, paperweights or bookends. For into each calcedony's core, millennia have poured alloyed amazement. A little technical assistance is frequently required for a calcedony to open up.

If you gaze within a calcedony's treasure crypt, you may find terraced fields of fertile laminations, beneath azure summer afternoon skies that float Styrofoam explosions of crystalline cloud. Later you may find shimmering mica skies that reflect sparkling seas of petrified stars.

Calcedonies are forged in many different rock formations and found all over the world. Depending on the culture in which the calcedony exists, it may endow wisdom or courage, healing powers or spiritual powers. Sometimes all of these, and in these ways, calcedonies contribute to the community in which they are found. Each calcedony is unique, wonderfully one of a kind.

Friends gave me calcedonies as gifts because they knew I loved them — calcedonies and them. Gifts like my agate pendant, whose polished cross-sectional slice of concentric rings in unimaginable shades of amber, rust, and gold, once dangled from my neck on an old black leather shoelace. I always wore that pendant, even in the shower. I don't anymore — wear my pendant or shower. I get immersion baths from time to time, though not as often as I would like, but the pendant disappeared a few years ago.

Another friend gave me my amethyst paperweight. An oyster shell–coloured crèche, sheltering shimmering clusters of purple spikes that emanate light, like in the first Superman movie. My amethyst paperweight held down my scraps of always-uncompleted poetry, so my always-thankopen window could always be open without scattering my thoughts beyond their always-then scattered state onto the floor or out the window. I have no idea where those paper scraps disappeared to, but I still have the poetry inside me waiting to burst out.

My bookends, though, are my favourite calcedonies. The friend who gave them to me said their coarse, crusty, outer surfaces reminded her of me. My bookends are beautiful. The outer surfaces are the speckled dull grey and brown they have been for billions of years, but their now-cut-open insides have been polished smooth and lacquered to bring out brilliant rainbows of chestnut and summer wheat and setting sun.

My bookends are so heavy that I used to work out with them, holding one in each hand and doing arm curls to grow strong muscles. Of course when I was using my bookends as dumbbells, my books frequently found themselves balanced precariously on my desk, or more than likely spread all over my desk. Sometimes spread all over the floor. The books my bookends bookended grew my mind much better than my bookends grew my biceps. But my bookends no longer bookend my books. Because my books ended. It has been seventeen years since I turned a page. I can no longer grow my brain with my books, or grow my muscles with my bookends for that matter.

I still have my bookends. They now bookend my computer, which sits on my desk instead of books. My computer waits there patiently for me to press its power button. And one day

I will press that power button. And when I do, the rainbow arcs of my bookends will truly become a rainbow over which my computer will fly me to a better-than-emerald place. A place from which I will never return.

At night, under the grey fluorescent light of my room in the group home where I live, each half of my bookends looks like a cross-section of a brain or a CT scan like you see on TV doctor shows: the crenulated outline of the "cerebral cortex," the dark of fluid in the "ventricles." My bookends' brain resemblance reminds me to mention that I have a neurological condition. Not that I need bookends to remind me, it's just a convenient cue to tell you that my brain no longer communicates with my muscles — any of my muscles — except those that open my eyes, move my eyeballs, breathe me, and, most important, move my jaw. My other muscles are totally incommunicado, put on ice, held in isolation, or whatever police-show slang you like.

My brain muscles, as you have gathered by now, work exceptionally well. Even my doctors think my brain muscles work exceptionally well, and doctors are *supposed* to have exceptional brain muscles so they would know. (I must emphasize the word *supposed* as sometimes I'm not so sure.) However, as doctors see the rest of my body as so unwell, they can't help but see my brain as exceptional. I guess it's better to have a "well-functioning" brain than a "well-functioning" body, I mean if you had to choose one or the other. Though sometimes I'm not so sure.

I know you can't wait to hear more about my amazing brain muscles, but first let me tell you about my amazing jaw muscles. They allow me to speak, albeit quietly and seldom heard. My jaw muscles allow me to eat, although an attendant at the group home has to shovel the food into my mouth before my jaw muscles can chew the food, which my jaws do quite well, thank-you-very-much. And most important, my jaw muscles work the joystick for my power chair, my powerful magic wand. My joystick is attached to the right armrest of my power chair and comes up and across to cup under my chin. All I have to do is move my jaw forward or from side to side, and my joystick engages the big batteries under my bum to propel me to joy.

From the moment I wake up each day, I can't wait to get my chin on my joystick. But I do wait. And wait. I have no choice but to wait. I have to patiently wait to be cleaned up, teeth brushed, hair brushed if I'm lucky, bum loaded into chair, head Velcro-strapped back to head support, joystick cup positioned under my chin, more Velcro to hold my head down to my joystick. Then I take a deep breath and bask in the sweet sensation of feeling my chin caress my joystick's smooth cup.

While I wait for someone to have time for the cleaning up and brushing and lifting and Velcroing, which I always hope will happen early in the morning and in an uninterrupted sequence but often happens late in the afternoon, I contemplate what adventures the day may bring. Because when the patient wait is finally over, my joystick frees me. At least to manoeuvre around the group home to the TV room, to the dining room, back to my bedroom. Although there's not much room for manoeuvring in the group home.

There is one place where, when no one is watching, I can actually dance. And you should see me dance. I dance my ass off, any chance I get. I dance to the records, eight tracks, and tapes that are always playing in my head: Stones, Kinks, Airplane. They don't make music like that anymore so I don't mind not being able to buy new stuff, or play it for that matter. I also waltz gracefully to "Unchained Melody," Righteous Brothers' version of course, and "This Nearly Was Mine" from Rodgers and Hammerstein's *South Pacific*. I also love slow dancing to more modern romantic stuff, like "Lady in Red" by Chris de Burgh. But my favourite music to dance to is, of course, Michael Jackson. I do a mean moonwalk to "Billie Jean." Believe me, Michael Jackson has nothing on me. I have to admit I even do some pretty smooth disco moves to Donna

Summer, Thelma Houston, and *Saturday Night Fever* Bee Gees. I love that movie, but of course would never admit it.

When I'm in hospital, that is after I've recovered enough from what got me there, my power chair has more room to pick up speed. Of course, bombing around in my chair in the hospital is only possible if someone has had the time to arrange putting my chair into a van so that it can join me in the hospital, and again only if someone in the hospital has had time to strap me into my chair. However, when the sun and the moon and the stars align, my power chair becomes a Formula 1 race car. My joystick is its accelerator pedal, clutch, and steering wheel combined, and my racing helmet is made from Velcro straps wrapped around my head to hold it against the car's headrest, complete with chinstrap.

I rev my engine, one foot on the accelerator, another on the brake, my right hand feeling the vibration of the gear shifter's knob, my left hand on the small steering wheel. I shift into gear and bomb down the halls at full throttle. I accelerate into 90° turns, of which there are many in hospitals, handling them smooth as silk, and when no nurses or receptionists are at a nursing station I even do hairpin turns around their counters, handling them with equal aplomb. When I enter a turn, my sharp eyes, behind my racing goggles, fix on the inside curb. My soft hands, in fire-resistant gloves of course, nimbly caress the wheel. Coming out of the turn, I quickly pick up some serious speed and head down the long straightaway, of which, again, there are many in hospitals. I can do zero to sixty in less than five seconds, and, if I'm lucky, I can pick off a doctor or two, sideswiping their kneecaps, unintentionally of course, or crashing them into a concrete wall. I've made a blood sport out of playing bumper cars with doctors' knees.

However, my favourite doctor blood sport is more *Blood and Sand* with Tyrone Power than *Winning* with Paul Newman, although I'm in love with Paul Newman's baby blues. When I spot a doctor down the hall, I hit the brakes on my chair, so

8   Patiently Waiting For ...

I can pause to savour the chaos I'm about to create. I stare down the hall at the doctor's white coat as if it were a matador's red cape. I slowly move my jaw left or right, turning my chair's front wheels to take aim at the matadoctor's white cape, taunting me, taunting me. Matadoctors are unaware of my capacity in my chair to challenge them and the conceptions they work within. My left foot stamps the sand of the bullring. I breathe in as deeply as I can, then snort menacingly. I breathe in even deeper, and snort, even more menacingly. After enough of these breathe-snort cycles to gush my adrenalin to ferocity level, I push my chin as forward as possible and charge at full speed at the matadoctor like a ferocious bull.

Doctors never notice me until I am almost upon them because patients in halls (and in waiting rooms for that matter) are invisible to doctors. So when a doctor finally sees me bearing down upon him, with no intention of swerving from my bloody course, surprise, shock, then terror grip his eyes before he quickly plasters himself against the nearest wall, or dodges into a patient's room, or into the elevator he's been waiting for if its doors open in time to save him. It's the most fun I ever have because doctors are the most chickenshit of toreadors.

It's also great feeling the eyes of nearby doctors, cautiously watching my back as I speed off. They're wondering how my chair can move that fast. And who gave me permission to drive so fast? And why I don't have more control of my chair? And better driving manners? And why am I even allowed in the halls of their "active treatment" palace? Or in their "active treatment" palace at all, using up its "scarce resources," rather than being in a "chronic care" facility where "chronics" like me belong?

So you can see why I love scaring the shit out of doctors. And I really do scare the shit out of some doctors. I know that as fact because my sense of smell still works, and I always take a quick sniff as I speed by. And of course I'm sensitive to the smell of shit, steeping in it as I do while patiently waiting for someone to clean me up. Not the most fragrant of teas.

Unlike matadors, matadoctors never beckon me to another charge. In fact they usually flee next time they see me. But just like matadors kill bulls, the matadoctors will kill me in the end. The crowd may even cheer.

Chapter 3

November 15, 1997

I know I promised to tell you about my brain, but first let me tell you just a little more about the rest of my body. I could be burned at the stake, like Ingrid Bergman in *Joan of Arc*, and feel no pain. That is, until my chin caught fire. The no-pain thing always amazes medical students when they come to practise their neurological exam skills on me. Of course, a neurological exam always includes the "pinprick test."

You don't know about the "pinprick test"? Then you're lucky. In a "pinprick test," a little prick — pricks your skin — with a little pin — to determine — which areas of your skin — can still send pain messages to your brain and which cannot. All medical students call these little areas of skin *dermatomes*. I call all medical students "little pricks," as I have no insight into any medical student's true prick size and believe in equality, and, of course, there are more women in medical school now than when I first became a voodoo doll. I call all medical students "little pricks" even when they're not pricking me.

If a medical student acts like an arrogant prick, I mess him up a bit. Like by pretending to wince in pain every time he pricks me. And if my whimpering doesn't stop the arrogant asshole, or at least cause him to genuinely apologize, I shriek "Fuck!" when the pin pricks me. Of course, I have to see their hand go down to predict when the pin pricks me, which has taken quite a while to perfect. It's a hoot watching them flinch back when I scream, apologizing profusely as they bolt from my bed. Some little pricks even shriek back. One even screamed "Fuck" back to me. And one little prick actually pricked himself. I actually felt sorry for that one and asked if he was bleeding. He took his finger out of his mouth to make sure he wasn't, but he actually was. He kept looking at his finger, then from his finger back to me and back to his finger, looking scared, until I said,

"C'mon big boy, I'm not infectious," which scared him more, as if he was now seriously considering the possibility.

Actually I'm fond of medical students. Really. Especially the ones who try to be confident and charming, but are so insecure they can't pull it off. Anyway, medical students are a great distraction. Sure help me bear the boredom. Okay, I really do like medical students but it's too bad they grow up to become doctors.

So you must be wondering by now why I'm in an active treatment hospital getting pricked. It's personal but I'll tell you anyway. I get pressure sores "down there." "Down there" being how doctors refer to the general area of a woman's body with parts that cannot be named in polite company. And I get pressure sores "down there" because we who cannot feel pressure "down there" cannot shift our weight off our "down theres" like you who can feel your "down theres" do all the time without realizing it. They sometimes call pressure sores "bedsores," though the bed doesn't get sore. It's the bed that causes you to get sore, or at least it would cause you to get sore if you could feel what the bed was doing. But if you could feel what the bed was doing, you'd turn your butt a bit to get the pressure off the skin, and then you wouldn't get bedsores. Not very complicated. Anyway, if you are a woman "like me," you can get bedsores "down there." And if a bedsore gets infected you get admitted to hospital for IV antibiotics. So here I am.

I once made one of the nurses show me what an infected bedsore looks like. Once was enough, thank-you-very-much. The nurse had to use two mirrors to show me a silver dollar–sized disc containing concentric thick circles of blackish-blue, red, and yellow crud, sort of an angry archery target, ragged and spewing rage. Once, one of my bedsores became so infected that the infection spread quickly throughout my body and almost killed me while I was still in the Emergency Department.

Women who get bedsores on our "private parts," another term used by doctors who don't want to offend our sensitive natures with bad manners, actually consider them "private parts" even though we go on public display several times a day for diaper changes, and sometimes also need changed the little catheter tube to our bladder that enters our body just below our clitoris and above our vagina. Sorry to have to name these private parts for geographical accuracy. So you would think that after all these years, I would get used to my private parts being exposed, but they're still private parts. I make private parts jokes when the nurses change my catheter; it lightens up the procedure. I get laughs from the nurses and caregivers who have been in Canada for a while. The more-recent-to-Canada caregivers, forever kind and polite, look at me sympathetically because they're sure my brain is now going the way of the rest of my body. By the way, rule number one for people "like me" is staying popular with the nurses and caregivers. Otherwise it's shit on you and urine on the floor, and you're breathing the fumes all day and, believe me, not getting high. And when I'm in hospital, I have the other patients in the ward to consider.

Chapter 4

February 6, 1998

A gurney slides by on my left. Without lifting my eyes from the thick stack of blood work results that have been patiently waiting for me on the counter of our Clinic's nurses' station, I see the gurney bears a woman, motionless. I have seen this woman before somewhere. As I flip through the blood result slips, scanning for any urgent highs or lows, I hear the gurney being bumped into one of our cramped examining rooms. I do not lift my eyes, even as the gurney's struggle through the exam room door clatters the two IV poles dangling three antibiotic bags. She must be infected somewhere. I hope she's on pain meds.

As is customary, the Chief Resident will assess the patient with our nurse first, while I remain at the nurses' station working my way through the test results and simultaneously dictating a consultation note on our previous patient. Before I'm halfway through the note, the Chief Resident opens the examining room door and curtly announces, "Ready." He is becoming a good technical surgeon, but I fear he has already become a too efficient physician. While the nurse and I are still entering the examining room, the Chief Resident starts presenting, in his machine-gun staccato abbreviations, what motivated the referral of the patient to our Team for consultation.

"Three-centimetre infected bedsore — ulcerating skin of vulva — south and to west of vagina — looks like hell — took swabs."

I gently close the door behind me.

He fires on, "Came in unconscious — through Emerg — three nights ago — total body sepsis — probably blood-spread infection from bedsore — on triple antibiotics — same we would use — still out of it — nothing more we can do for bedsore — or for her for that matter — quadriplegic."

Quadriplegic. I knew I have seen this woman before. In fact, I have seen her several times over the year, racing down our Hospital's halls in her electric wheelchair. I was amazed at how fast she could move that thing. And they must be hard to control because she almost plowed me over a couple of times.

Now that I see her still for the first time, I see dark eyes, slightly visible through heavy eyelids and thick eyebrows. I see dishevelled black hair, clinging damply to her forehead, with wisps of grey at her temples. I see thin lips drawn down at the left corner of her mouth, the drinking-straw lips of chronic infirmity. I see a small, frail body beneath the hospital-white sheets.

I ask the Chief Resident to start again, this time assuming our patient is fully awake.

"But we're not in the operating room," he quips.

This is supposed to be a joke, as I am derided for insisting that all operating room personnel treat my anaesthetized patients as if they are awake. I have insisted this ever since I was Chief Resident, when just as I was about to paint an anaesthetized patient's abdomen with Proviodine antiseptic for the surgical incision, I noticed she had written on her abdomen in black magic marker "NO FAT JOKES PLEASE." The ink was so indelible that it did not come off when I scrubbed her abdomen with the Proviodine.

I do not acknowledge the Chief Resident's quip; I just stare at the woman's slightly open eyes.

The Chief Resident impatiently says, "She really can't hear us, I tried." Then he shouts at her, "Do you know where you are?" and claps his hands an inch above her face.

She does not respond.

I ask the Chief Resident to introduce our patient to me as if she is awake.

He says, "We're going to be late for the OR."

I keep staring at her eyes.

He utters an exaggerated sigh. "All right, this is Mrs. or Miss _____."

"I would prefer her first name please."

He looks at the chart. "Ruth."

"Hello, Ruth. I'm sorry you're not feeling well."

I say this softly to eyes that seem to be staring back at me. Full of understanding. She does not respond.

"It is important that I examine the bedsore on your vulva even though Dr. ____ has already examined it."

She does not respond.

The Chief Resident responds with a mock gasp and "Don't you trust me" look. Then he reminds me that, "They will be waiting to start our case in the OR soon, and you told me to remind you that we don't want to be late again."

I stare at the patient's eyes.

"Ruth, I know you are not able to speak to me, but if you can hear me, can you twitch one of your facial muscles, perhaps your lips."

She does not respond.

"You may not be able to give me permission to examine you, but it is very important that I examine your bedsore."

I stare at the patient's eyes.

"The nurse and I are going to drape you, and lift your knees in a way that will expose your bedsore. We will keep you as covered as possible."

She does not respond.

The nurse helps me pull up the white sheet to position it below the patient's knees. We gently lift her emaciated calf muscles upward and outward to the frog leg position. I part the white curtains to see a three-centimetre jagged circle of blackened skin, screaming skin. The central part of the lesion exhibits the red rage of infection with a purulent yellow ooze dripping from its core like tired tears. I touch the skin surrounding the lesion to determine how deep the infection extends. Deep. I close the drapes.

I say to myself, "I hope the antibiotics can ameliorate the infection. I don't think surgery is the answer."

I say to the patient, in the muted doctor's tones she has probably heard many times before, what she has heard so many times before, "I am sorry, but there is nothing more we can do."

Perhaps it is her dignity, engaging me through her barely open eyes after my objective observation of her private wound. Perhaps it is her understanding, compelling me through her vertical brow crease. Perhaps it is her tranquility, eloquently speaking to me through her unmoving lips. Perhaps it is all of these that move me to take her hospital chart from the Chief Resident's hands. His "what are you doing?" glare reminds me how rare it is for me to hold a patient's chart.

I open the thick manila cardboard cover, lined front and back with numerous dates of admission, and flip to an amber "Request for Consultation" sheet near the back. I carefully read the note from the Internal Medicine Resident, then the quickly scribbled response beneath written by our Chief Resident before he called me into the examining room. He has it right, nothing more to do than hope the high-dose antibiotics take control of the infection.

Then, for some strange reason, I flip back the many pages of the patient's chart to the first page. Her date of birth and mine are identical: same year, same month, same day. I am transfixed.

The Chief Resident tries to interrupt my stare with, "Should I call the OR and tell the anaesthetist not to put your patient to sleep?"

Without moving my eyes from our birthdate, I whisper, "Please go down to the OR and apologize to my patient for me.

Please explain to her that I am unavoidably delayed and will be down in a few minutes."

"Are you sure?"

"Then apologize to the nurses for me, and the anaesthetist." I hear him quickly leave and close the door harshly.

My eyes rivet the hundreds of haunting pages.

Chapter 5

November 15, 1997

I was an artist before I went from "able-bodied" to chin-bodied, from free spirit to — well I'm still a free spirit, but could easily be much freer if I could just fucking get my joystick connected to my computer. Sorry about that. Anyway, I went to art school out of high school and learned a lot there, like I couldn't draw worth shit and instructors are paid to make you keep trying, which I did. But I found drawing too confining. I much preferred working with colour and shape and texture with thick gobs of oil paint rather than skinny pencils or charcoal sticks. I also liked pottery, particularly working with the glazes. I was amazed each post-kiln day by the abstract beauty the glazes had baked on my clay pots.

Soon after my diagnosis, I left art school to tramp around Europe while I still could tramp. Travelling Europe was great of course, but I had my heart set on being an artist, and a different type of biological clock was ticking in me that was becoming more and more difficult to ignore. So I returned.

I thought I could support myself best as a potter. Earthy-looking pots were in because everyone was emulating the new species called Earth Mamas, eager to discard their delicate department-store bone china from Japan, frilly trimmed cups and bowls and all, in favour of the warmth, weight, and originality of locally produced, one-of-a-kind clay coffee mugs and fruit bowls.

So I got a waitressing job to support myself becoming a potter. My first tips would be gloriously exchanged for a clay-firing kiln. I got a job at an upscale restaurant, figuring more revenue there. My face hurt from its constant plastic smile, my most sparkling smile I might add, and my knees hurt from the expected, albeit intermittent, genuflecting of subservience. But the tips came slower than I had hoped and my muscles weakened faster than I, and the doctors, had expected.

Dawdling my way to work one day along a sunny sidewalk brimming with kiosks, I saw a beautiful necklace of colour-dazzled copper enamel pieces. Each piece was a unique shape, and the enamel on each piece had melted into totally original designs and hues. These complex pieces of art were strung together by a simple black leather shoelace thing.

If I worked in copper enamel, I wouldn't have to lift those heavy bags of wet clay anymore. And I bet a copper-enamelling kiln would be much cheaper than a clay-baking kiln, as less heat would probably be required to melt the enamel bits on copper than to bake clay, and the copper-enamelling kiln would probably be much smaller. That day, I went to price a copper-enamelling kiln, and sure enough I had enough tip money saved to write a cheque for my kiln right on the spot. The next day I started creating art for a living. I made necklaces, earrings, pendants, bracelets. You name it. I wasn't going to become rich, but I was an artist. Goes with the territory, so to speak.

I poured all of me into copper enamelling. I developed a special relationship with my kiln. He was very much my partner in creating jewellery. Yes my kiln is a "he." His name is Fred. Fred has supernatural powers. Fred melted the enamel pieces on my shaped copper pieces in his very skilled and special way, resulting in art that I could never even imagine, let alone accomplish. Fred's talent came from his ability to set each coloured enamel bit free to create, each bit having room both for its own artistic expression and to work with the other enamel pieces to integrate and blend their colours and shapes to create complex art that no single bit of enamel, nor any human, could have created by itself. It was as if I were providing little copper canvases for Fred and the enamel bits to create their own art. Fred was so very much my partner that the sign on my studio read "Jewellery by Fred and Ruth."

When I got moved into my first chronic care "facility," I had to sell what furniture and kitchen things I had, and give away most of my clothes, even my books. But I couldn't give Fred away. I asked a friend to keep him for me just in case some new treatment came along that would allow Fred and me to create again. She said she would store him in her garage. I haven't spoken to her for years but Fred might still be there, patiently waiting for me.

I know I should give Fred away to someone as a gift. To someone who can use Fred's gift. And I know I will give Fred away one day, but that day will be after I start creating again. You see, I will start creating again. Just not with copper enamel and Fred. I will create again with my computer and we will write poetry together. If they will only fucking hook me up to my computer. "We have the technology" as they say at the beginning of *The Six Million Dollar Man*.

Let me tell you about my computer. It's a Mac. Apple developed disability-friendly software years ago. When I heard about it, I cashed in my savings and bought a real beauty. My computer looks like it won first prize for design at some arty high-tech college. Its ultra modern yet practical structure glows in a sparkling pearl finish, even when my computer is not turned on. Actually, my computer has never been turned on, so I have lots of time to admire the elegance of its design. But I didn't blow my wad to stare at an aesthetically pleasing desk ornament. I want to use my computer like other people do and, of course, to write poetry.

One day I will turn my computer on. My jaw will operate my computer through my joystick in the same way your hand pushes the power button and operates a mouse. Only I won't need a mouse pad. Apple's "disability-friendly platform" will be my rocket-launching pad, and I will blast off from my current world and never re-enter.

I ordered my Apple with a new voice-activated software program already installed. It's called "Dragon." Really. You don't believe me? I swear on my chin it's called "Dragon." "Dragon" will allow words to flame from my mouth and appear on my computer screen, not to mention the screens of people all over the world. "Dragon" will allow me to talk with these people, share thoughts with these people, learn from these people. And, most important, "Dragon" will allow me to finally write my poems, so many poems, poems I have collected in my heart for so many years.

I once asked a caregiver if she would write down a few lines of a poem I was trying to write in my head. She actually said "Yes," and actually returned to my room during her break. But, it didn't work out. It was hard for me to fully conceive the poem in my head before I spoke it to her, and when I tried to speak a few lines off the top of my head, it was embarrassing, because the lines were not fully baked yet, not ready to be heard. And I felt rushed because I was using up this kind caregiver's precious break time, and considering their breaks are so short, time she was taking from other inmates and from her other chores. And my poems are personal.

If I could only be connected to my computer, I would speak a line and see the words appear on the screen. Then, over time, I would add more words when they move me and move the words around until they convey what I feel. I would spend all day gently massaging the words as the words gently massage me. Once my computer comes alive and starts helping me write poems, I will of course call my computer Fred.

However, a bi-o-me-di-cal engineer is required to calibrate my jaw muscles with my computer's computations. To interface my face with my computer's face, so to speak. I have been on the waiting list for a bi-o-me-di-cal engineer to hook me up for over a year now. I was told it would be about a three-year wait, because there are only two bi-o-me-di-cal engineers in our "region." Can you imagine that there would be only two bi-o-me-di-cal engineers who can connect the umbilical cords of people "like me," people who need to be connected to be able to communicate with people "like you," and "like me." And apparently no more bi-o-me-di-cal engineers can be hired because of the government's fucking clawbacks to funding healthcare and social services. Sorry about that again.

So I wait for the engineer, addling my brain on the TV shows that come up on the last channel someone had time to turn to for me. Another two years is a long time to wait, knowing that the day I get hooked up to my computer will be the first day of my beautiful new life; knowing that I'm probably running out of time for a beautiful new life. But I must wait. I must be patient and wait.

Chapter 6

February 7, 1998

I stand outside the door to her room, the evening following my consultation. "Visitors' hours are now over" has been announced three times in the woman's voice that I have heard so many times over the years, so I know it is well past nine o'clock. I have been at this door twice before in the past hour, but both times retreated to my office two floors up. I have tried to stay in my office, convincing myself that I should be working on revisions to a research paper due this week. I have tried to go home, knowing that if I left now, I could kiss my children "Goodnight," like I try to do every night, but too often fail to do. However, I am again drawn to this door.

I need to know more about her. Not medically, for I have withdrawn from her care. I have never before ended a doctor–patient relationship, but I knew that if I was to learn more about her, this was required. Required ethically. So I formally asked one of my colleagues to do any follow-up consultations if she was again referred to our service. I even wrote a note in her chart to further formalize the termination of our doctor–patient relationship and the transfer of her care.

I have ended my doctor–patient relationship with her to dissolve the power differential inherent in the doctor–patient relationship. Dissolving this relationship is ethically essential because I hope to be able to ask her to tell me things about herself that are not related to her current clinical problem, the problem for which I was consulted. I want to know her story beyond the medical story stored in inscribed snippets on two-holed paper, held together by bent metal fasteners in her thick hospital chart. I want to learn her desires for the present, her hopes for her future.

This need to know more about a patient than I require for objective clinical care is definitely not like me, and indeed not like any physician I know. But she has been on my mind constantly, and I need to speak with her, apologize to her, learn from her. So I lean on the wall outside of her door, admonishing my presence here as "inappropriate," calling myself "ridiculous."

I take a deep breath and courage myself to enter her room. It is a four-bed ward, dimly lit by upward-facing fluorescent grey lights fixed to the wall over each bed. A monitor of some sort beeps beside one of the two beds on my left, as I enter. Both beds are demarcated by drawn curtains; the pastel blue, pink, and tan plaid curtains with fishnet borders on top seemed so advanced and modern when I started working here. The first bed on my right is empty. Her bed is in the far right corner. It is not curtained off.

I walk tentatively to the foot of her bed. The translucent skin of her face displays the television program running silently on the hospital TV, suspended from a stand above her bed like a hanging head. It is hard to distinguish precisely the characteristics of her face amidst the creeping colours and flickering shapes on her skin. Her eyes seem shut. The arms of the TV's audio set pincer her ears like a stethoscope. She looks like she is listening to the heartbeat of the TV. She must no longer be comatose. It would be unlikely for a TV to be set up for a comatose patient, although probably not a bad idea. The antibiotics must be working. She must be sleeping.

Suddenly I feel like a voyeur. I quickly turn to leave, but decide to shut off the television so that she can sleep more peacefully. I push the red-lit power button on the TV's lower left corner. The TV's screen cones down to a white dot and goes black. Her face is peaceful without the television's interference. I turn to leave, but decide that she would sleep more peacefully without the audio set in her ears. I quickly bend over her face, and gently remove the pieces from her ears. I straighten up quickly and hit my head on the television. I quickly move the TV farther away from her face, and run out of the room.

I lean against the wall beside her door, where I had been leaning just a few minutes before, again taking deep breaths, again admonishing myself. Suddenly my shirt soaks in cold sweat as I realize my stupid mistake. What if she should wake up in the night? She will not be able to turn the television back on. Nor will she be able to press the call button to request a nurse come in to turn it back on for her. She will just stare at the dark screen because of my stupidity, my misplaced assistance. How ignorant can I be?

I run back to her bed, and move the television back to where I think it was before I moved it. I turn the TV on. I start to go, but remember the stethoscope. I hurry to separate the audio set's arms and place its earpieces back into her ears. I run out of the room and up the stairs to my office. I collapse on my couch, trying hard to catch my breath.

Chapter 7

February 8, 1998

I have developed another bedsore. This one got infected, really infected, and the infection spread throughout my body to become a-total-sepsis-of-my-body. Don't worry, the "big gun" antibiotics are killing the little buggers, and I'm feeling much better today thank-you-very-much. But this particular infected bedsore really scared me because of how quickly the infection spread. It spread so quickly that by the time the caregiver found me and the ambulance got me to Emerg — wait — I'll have to tell you about that later because some strange doctor has just come into my room. Well he's almost come into my room. He seems to be glued to the floor in the doorway. He's staring at me though. That's never good.

Now he's walking over to my bed. Now he's stuck to the floor again, staring at me several feet away from the foot of my bed. Staring very strangely I might add. Staring at my eyes. Doctors never spend this much time looking directly into a patient's eyes, unless they're an ophthalmologist and protected by some instrument or another and very well paid to look into your eyes, of course. It's getting really strange at the foot of my bed.

"I am no longer your physician."

He says this in a very slow, very deep voice, sort of like God talking to Moses in *The Ten Commandments*. Except he added "no longer," and used the word "physician" instead of God, although they probably are synonymous terms to him, like most doctors.

So I take my time and carefully choose my first words to him.

"Who — the — fuck — are — you?"

But as I'm still weak from my total body sepsis, "fuck" comes out quieter than my usual, and as he's a doctor, and probably has never heard a patient use the "F" word before, let alone when directly referring to him, he's not sure he hears me right. Or he can't believe he hears me right. Or is just stunned.

Then his expression starts to change. He's starting to look flustered, even frightened. He keeps looking at the door like he wants to leave. But instead he takes a chair belonging to the empty bed beside mine, places it close to the head of my bed, puts his white-coated bony ass on it, and leans his head over my face so his right ear is close to my lips.

I repeat as loudly as I can, "Who — the — fuck — are — you?"

This time I know he hears me because he jerks bolt upright, hitting the back of his head on the TV, which normally would have pissed me off because a nurse had positioned it just right, then he sits back down. He turns his head to longingly look at the door again. I think he's preparing to bolt through it. He glances back at me, then back at the door again and back at me and back at the door. He's obviously plotting his escape. Then he stares at me, and stares at me, and stares at me, and stares at me. Finally, he looks down at his feet and says,

"I'm sorry."

I pretend not to hear him. He probably thinks I'm hard of hearing. Most doctors think quads are hard of hearing on top of everything else we've got going. But actually not being able to hear him is quite reasonable because I have the TV set's earpieces plugged into my ears. However they're just hospital-issue jobbies and don't block out any hospital noise including his. I just stare back at him.

He lifts his head and looking directly at me speaks very slowly and loudly with his lips mouthing the words as if he's sure I need to lip-read, "I'm sorry."

I usually straighten docs out when they speak slowly and loudly at me, but I decide to give this guy a break because there is the slim possibility that he sees that my ears are plugged and doesn't want to take the plugs out, and assumes I can lip-read because my ears are almost always plugged into TV earpieces when in hospital.

So I say in my best Maggie Smith Miss Jean Brodie, "Dear boy, could you be a darling and unplug my ears, thank-you-very-much?"

He hesitates and starts to get up, very carefully, watching out for the TV. He awkwardly bends over me, still watching out for the TV. His hands remain at his sides. He just stares at the audio plugs, as if taking them out of my ears requires a well-thought-out strategy and surgical precision. Finally, he slowly reaches his hands out toward each side of my face. He hesitates there, and then very gingerly separates the arms of the audio set, careful not to touch my ears or other parts of my face for that matter.

Having accomplished this feat, he quickly straightens up, banging the back of his head on my TV and, of course, moving it further out of place.

"Now what's that you were saying, dear boy?" Still in Maggie Smith.

"I'm sorry, I'm Doctor —"

"Sorry," I swiftly cut him off. "Is your name Dr. Sorry or are you sorry you're a doctor?" I'm keeping up the Maggie Smith, like I do when I meet any new doctor so they think I'm a wealthy British woman and will be polite to me because of my social standing, proper upbringing, and finishing-school education. There's also the hope they'll even give more time to my care as I understand doctors do for wealthy, well-schooled patients.

"No. Neither," he mumbles.

"So if you're not Dr. Sorry, and you're not sorry you're a doctor — which you should be, by the way, dear boy — what then? What the fuck is your name?"

He's frozen stiff, staring his shocked eyes into my calm as always eyes.

He keeps staring. I better back off the swearing before I cause him serious harm.

Finally he blurts out, "I'm Dr. ____."

Let's leave out his name to protect the guilty.

Then he says, "May I speak with you for a few minutes?" almost pleading.

"Well, Doc, I may just happen to have some free time in my crowded social calendar today because my yoga class was cancelled. Let me check."

He stares again. I think he's trying to ignore what I just said, or at least not think about what I just said. Or maybe everything I've said has sort of blown his mind and it's taking him a while to put the pieces back in.

"I want to apologize to you."

"You should apologize, Doc. It's late and I need my beauty sleep if I'm ever going to get paid big bucks to hump a pole again."

Open mouth again. He's staring at my eyes, afraid to look lower than my chin. He keeps staring. Finally he stands at attention and, missing the TV, plods onward.

"I came to see you last night but you were sleeping."

"You know, Doc, that is what people do at night, even quads."

He's shaking his head trying hard to ignore what I say so he can get on with what he's come to say. It's as if he's memorized a carefully written speech, and he's worried he'll miss something if I keep interrupting him. So, of course, I interrupt him again.

"And why would a man come to see a woman late at night when she's sleeping?"

No response.

"You're not tall enough to be Christopher Lee."

He doesn't smile, probably has no idea who Christopher Lee is so I give him a clue.

"And your teeth aren't nearly big enough."

He's probably never ever seen *Horror of Dracula*. Or any other vampire flick. Doctors don't go to the movies, or watch TV, for that matter. I'm wasting my breath not to mention my wit on him.

"Okay, Doc, get on with it."

"I'm here to apologize to you for watching the colours of your television set reflect on your face while you were sleeping last night."

Now I'm the one who's staring, but I quickly recover with, "Doc, if you were that interested in what was on TV you could've turned the TV around to watch it."

Stunned look again. No sense of humour. No doctors have a sense of humour. But, get this, after watching my face for a bit, he — and these are his exact words — "felt like a voyeur" because he says it was wrong of him to look at my face "without my permission." So he decided to leave.

I'm staring at him again trying to figure out how strange a doctor can be and still be allowed to be a doctor, but he's not finished yet.

"I also want to apologize to you for examining you without your permission in a non-emergency, albeit urgent, situation."

"What? When?"

"When you were unconscious."

"And exactly what part of me did you examine without my permission?"

"I examined the bedsore on your vulva."

"Whoa, whoa, whoa, Doc."

I really thought doctors couldn't say anything to throw me off anymore. So of course I make him explain in great detail what a "VULVA" is, insisting on all the anatomical and functional details. I then ask him to describe in precise detail what exactly did he do to my "VULVA."

Let me summarize: he looked at my crotch, and, yes, he probably touched my crotch, or at least one of his lackeys did, and "took swabs" from the bedsore on my crotch. I clearly must have been out of it, because these are the sorts of things a gal remembers, even if she can't feel her "VULVA."

He then says he hoped that I might have been able to hear him when he asked my permission to examine me, and his apology when he told me he was going to go ahead and examine me without my permission because there was no substitute decision-maker on my chart.

I quickly say, "No way, José," but by the time José is out of my mouth, I seem to remember something weird like a doctor telling another doctor to call me by my name. Maybe he did apologize to me for having to look at my bedsore without my permission. I'm not sure, but I don't tell him any of this, of course. I need to think about whether he'd feel worse if I did hear him ask permission to examine my VULVA and I did not give him my permission, or would he feel worse if I did not hear him ask permission. Of course, I have to also decide how bad I want to make this nutbag feel. Probably very bad. But I need to think about it some more. And it looks like I'm going to have lots of time to think about it, because he's rambling on about being glad I don't remember him because he doesn't want "any vestige of doctor–patient relationship to exist." Yes, he really used the word *vestige*. Can you believe it? I let him mumble on about other nonsense, until I just can't take it any longer.

"Enough, Doc, enough. Stop. Why — are — you — here?"

He looks hurt but at least he shuts up.

"I'm here because I want to ask your permission to visit you in a non-medical capacity."

This guy's too weird.

He starts up the consent-shit rapid-fire again, "You're free to say no. Or, if you say yes now, you can change your mind at any time. You can take all the time you require to consider what I am asking, and please provide your permission only if you want to, and only when you're ready to." He stops but I think it's only because he has finally run out of breath.

He's asking my permission in such a formal way that I'm surprised he doesn't shove a consent form in my face, and put a pen in my hand to sign it. Not that he wouldn't have, if I could have.

He starts up again, rattling on about how he's already asked another doctor to follow up with my care, actually wrote a note on my chart, "formally dissolving our physician–patient relationship" so that he could approach me "as a potential friend." He says that "dissolving the doctor–patient relationship is important because of the large power differential that exists between physicians and their patients."

I'm suspicious of his motives and sure of his strangeness.

"Okay, Doc, enough. Why would you possibly want to visit me as my friend, when, if you stay my doctor, you can bill the system for visiting me. Even bill double for a Sunday night like tonight."

He tries to speak but stops, then he tries again in an almost defeated voice, "I just want to get to know you."

Sounds like a song title but I decide to give him a break. "Okay, Doc, you can visit me tonight since you're already here and in a non-medical way, whatever that means, because there's a slim chance you're better than boredom."

He gushes *thank you* over and over and so enthusiastically that he's embarrassing himself, which he clearly must do frequently. But I worry that a nurse might be listening to this from the hall, and being nice to a doctor might be interpreted as me getting soft, which would be bad for my reputation. So I stop him.

"But no looking at my VULVA anymore."

That stopped him. His mouth is open but I don't think he's breathing.

"Although I must have one hell of a VULVA."

He's frozen solid in stunness. A regular docsicle.

"Don't you agree Doc?"

I think I've put him into a hypnotic trance. Now I can get the truth out of him.

"Look deeply into my eyes. Deeply into my eyes. Now, Doc, tell me really why you want to visit me but not as my doctor."

He's still frozen.

"C'mon, Doc, the whole truth and nothing but."

Still frozen.

"Earth to strange Doc."

I'm starting to get worried that I stroked him out or something, so I give him in my best Cheech Marin, "You can do it. You can do it, Doc. The truth, why are you here?"

He quickly blurts out, "We are the same age."

"So what?"

"I mean we are exactly the same age. We were born same year, same month, same day."

This is getting *Twilight Zone* so I do the "Doo-doo-doo-doo, doo-doo-doo-doo" tune. He looks at me as if I am the one who's spaced out. Can you believe this guy? Then it hits me.

"You actually know my birthdate, Doc. Which means that you must have actually looked at my chart as well as my VULVA."

Same stunned look again.

"Only nurses, medical students, and residents ever look at a patient's chart. And as for VULVAS —"

Still stunned.

"Let's have another sign of life, Doc."

"Yes," he mumbles.

"Yes, you looked at my VULVA or at my chart?"

"Yes."

"Both?"

"Yes."

He's like a frozen robot that can only open his mouth to say, "Yes."

"Yes, both, I guess."

"You guess? That's not saying much for my VULVA."

"Yes."

"Here I thought it was of some interest to you."

"Yes."

"Well let me ask you a very easy question this time, Doc. Did you ever look at a patient's chart before? I assume you've looked at VULVAS before."

He's still frozen and I decide to leave him there for a while because I need time to think. Being born the same day has somehow connected this guy with me, probably in a there-but-for-the-grace-of-God-go-I way. I think this guy wants to know me because he feels sorry for me. And he feels sorry for me because he thinks I've had a tougher shake in life than him, identical birthdates and all. He feels sorry for me because he can walk, use his arms, etc. He doesn't understand that sympathy is the last thing I want. They don't teach important stuff like that in medical school.

I better get him going again. "Snap out of it, Doc."

This may again have been a mistake because he starts jabbering again at a feverish pace, telling me that he wants to know me "as a person not a patient," that he wants me to know him "as a person not a physician," that he wants to learn from me anything I "choose to share," anything that would help him understand my position, which is so different from his "even though we are exactly the same age," that he will "gratefully reciprocate" by telling me anything I want to know about him. Then he starts gasping as if he almost drowned. He keeps taking deep breaths and in between quietly says that he wants to be my "friend," to learn from me as a "friend," to learn for himself, to learn for his students.

Aha! The students. The ulterior motive. The medical students. Always the medical students. He wants his medical students to come and practise on me. He's just another arrogant, asshole doctor. Never trust a doctor. But he did have me going for a while.

He gets up and turns to leave, but it's been a boring day so I keep it going.

"Okay, Doc, what do you want 'to learn'?"

He asks me again to tell him "everything" about myself, "anything," "everything." Of course, instead of telling him anything about myself, I tell him everything about his lousy healthcare system and where he can shove it, but I'm not recovered enough yet to do justice to what I want to say so I stop.

He says, "You must be exhausted." He quickly stands and says, "Goodnight."

He's the one who's exhausted. You can tell by the way he's dragging himself to the door. He stops and turns back.

"Ruth, the TV's headset in your ears makes you look like you are wearing a stethoscope, listening to the TV's heartbeat."

Interesting. Maybe there's hope for this guy. So I give him in my best Rocky voice, "Yo, Doc, if you're not too busy tomorrow, drop in after work." I know, but he's better than boredom.

"I'd love to, but tomorrow is Monday," he says in a really apologetic voice.

"Monday, no kidding, Doc? You think quads don't know the days of the week?"

Stunned look again.

"On Monday nights, I facilitate an elective course for our medical students."

"An 'elective' course. Are you teaching your students to elect politicians who care about people, not just getting re-elected?"

"An elective means that the students are not required to attend."

"No kidding, Doc."

"Students who want to come, come but most of the guys stay home to watch Monday Night Football."

"Does that mean women become better doctors?"

"Sorry, I really have to go."

He quickly leaves. Very strange guy. Strange even for a doctor.

What does he really want from me? Maybe has some medical experiment in mind and he's being nice to me in the name of medical science. I bet he'll soon ask me to volunteer to get injected with some new experimental drug, tested previously only on animals. He probably thinks I would be a good candidate for research because he thinks I have nothing to lose. Maybe he's being nice to me so I will give him my permission to dissect part my brain after I die for research purposes, or even before I die, like the neurosurgeon wanted to do to John Travolta in *Phenomenon*. Nah, I'm not a phenomenon. There are too many women like me for him to see me as a phenomenon. And the surgery this guy performs is at the other end of things from a neurosurgeon, so to speak.

No, it's the sympathy bullshit that has him here on Sunday night.

Well, I've got news for you, Doc. Sympathy is not what I need. I need to be able to use my computer and I need a fucking biomedical engineer to hook my chair's joystick up to my computer so I can use it. Simple as that, Doc.

Chapter 8

May 6, 2000

I sit amidst a Circle of Friends
Friends who I had not previously met
Friends who know her
Though how well I cannot presume
Friends who do not know me
Or I would not have been invited
Friends who ought not be my friends.

The circle is really two semicircles
Facing each other
With spaces at each end
To enter the circle.
Eight women about her age
About my age
Sit silently in metal folding chairs
All sit pensively
All sit spiritually.
All are remembering her
All are celebrating her
All are finding comfort in this Circle of Friends
All except me.

Simple windows pour pastel rainbows
On the silent Circle
The windows' art
Melts with her art

On each of the women
While I struggle to avoid
The windows' warm paint.

All eyes are open
Reflecting peacefully
All hearts are open
Embracing her life
All hearts except my heart
Fixed in the formaldehyde of her death
Guilty of friendship denied.

"We would like you to come to our meeting,"
I was invited on the phone.
"It will be a simple memorial."
I said that I was sorry but had "another commitment."
"We would appreciate it if you could be with us."
I apologized again
"I have to be at a son's soccer game."

"It will be only a short meeting."
I apologized again
But knew that this was a meeting from which
My commitment to my children
Or my patients
Or my students
Could not exonerate me.

Ignoring my declines of her invitation she continued,
"You might share a few words."
I apologized again.
"But only if you want to."
I apologized again.
Even if it was possible for me to attend
It would not be possible for me to speak.

Chapter 9

February 9, 1998

He hurries into the hospital's main lecture theatre, seconds before he's scheduled to begin. He sees me right away. He has no choice. My chair is directly in front of the main doors, the only wheelchair-accessible entrance to this massive high-tech amphitheatre, and then there are steps going up. No ramps anywhere. So I'm stuck right here in front, feeling the eyes of the more than a hundred medical students behind me staring at the back of my chair and top of my head, and as they're used to doing, trying to figure out what I have.

I can tell he wants to start his class but he just keeps staring at me. I bet he's wondering how I got a doctor to write the order for me to leave the ward so soon after being so septic. Of course, no order was ever written. And wondering how I know where the amphitheatre is. Over the years, I've been displayed here by doctors many times for the benefit of medical students. He may even be wondering who pressed the elevator buttons for me, and who opened the doors to this part of the hospital. It's easy to get medical students to do what you want them to do. You just have to appear to know more than them, which is easy.

He forces his stare away from me and smiles at his students, who are also trying to force their stare away from me, but stare at me anyway, still looking for clues to what the patient has. Of course they can't help but see me as a patient: hospital-gowned, half-filled piss bag beside my chair's left wheel, no movement of limbs, head supported front and back. They're thinking the patient must have an "interesting" disease. After all, only patients with "interesting" diseases are presented in the hospital's largest lecture hall, and they've seen many other "interesting" patients here, albeit in regular business hours, on whom the doctor-lecturers demonstrate "interesting physical signs" of disease. So what does this patient have? Car accident quads are not "interesting" enough for a large lecture theatre. Maybe she has a "neurodegenerative disorder." Too many of them, so maybe a rare "variant" of a "neurodegenerative disorder." The students are also trying to figure out what test they want to ask the doctor to perform on the patient because he will soon ask them for suggestions to test her neurological connections, or lack thereof. Maybe they'll ask him to hit her knee with his "Queen Square hammer," and stick pins into her flesh.

The strange doctor's feet come even closer to mine, so he's sure I can see him. He thanks me for coming and tells me, "You're looking very well tonight."

Give me a break.

Then he quickly asks, "May I have your permission to introduce you to my students?"

What's with this guy and "permission"?

"And I want your permission to introduce you, as my friend, rather than as a patient here."

"Why not introduce me as someone born the same day as you?"

He starts to speak but stops. He's just staring at me again. I know he's late starting his class now, and really wants to get going, but what the heck.

"Hey Doc, what do you think of my slippers?"

He looks down at my furry bear paw slippers, complete with black felt claws. He's just about to say something, probably tell me how much he likes my slippers when I interrupt him with, "I've had these for years."

He freezes again, this time with his mouth open. He's trying to decide whether I am making a joke, because slippers do not wear out if you don't walk on them, or am I innocently applauding the hospital staff for not losing them. Me, innocent? Or am I trying to throw him off his carefully thought-out introduction to tonight's "exploration?" Would I do such a thing? Or am I just trying to double-take him, or make him smile? I certainly did double-take him but he's not smiling.

Finally he forces his face to work. He's fumbling as he welcomes his students, and fumbling more as if he's trying to remember something, maybe how he had planned to introduce tonight's topic. He then takes a deep breath, looks at me, then at the students, smiles, and says, "We have a guest with us tonight, my friend, Ruth."

Chapter 10

February 9, 1998

I have to get by the nurses' station to make it safely back to my room. Neither tiptoeing nor mufflering my chair is a possibility, so I 180 my chair and nonchalantly back up slowly bedside the nurses' station so that the nurses, probably focused frenetically on their charting as usual, will think that I've just left my room to go for a stroll around the floor. But I am intercepted by the charge nurse, who snuck up behind me, and formally interrogates as to where I've been and what I've been up to. I am told that they've been looking all over the hospital for me, inside and out, and were just about to announce a "Code Yellow" over the hospital's PA system. I again promise never to leave the ward without permission again.

The charge nurse has already carefully documented my disappearance on my chart and now is writing again on my chart, this time that I again have promised never to leave the ward without permission. This is a game the charge nurses and I play so that the staff are not to blame for whatever may happen to me on one of my famous "walkabouts." I, of course, never make such promises, as I refuse to prostrate myself before the pen of permission of a doctor or the charge nurse who carries out his orders. I would rather remain a fixture on the ward like a toilet than beg permission from anyone. So I just leave the floor whenever it suits me.

When the formal interrogation and reprimand are finally finished, I am lifted back into bed. They notice that my piss bag is about to burst like a balloon, so they move quickly and I think I hear messily, to dispose of it and screw on a fresh one. My teeth are brushed, the TV channel is turned to the one I have calculated to have the fewest bad shows till I fall asleep, the headset is plugged into my ears. So now I finally have time to tell you what the medical students got tonight.

After very clumsily, almost incoherently, introducing the topic to be explored, the strange doctor-who-wants-to-be-my-friend asked for "volunteers" to be tonight's readers. Seven students, all women, went to the front and formed a semicircle, clearly having done this before. The student on the farthest left facing the audience stood directly in front of my feet, and turned to me slightly, actually facing me more than the audience. Then she began to read. The student-volunteers took turns reading from a poem by this Czech or German guy. I can't remember how the strange doctor put his nationality, but the poem was about a dwarf. But it was really about what it feels like to be different when people see "normal," in a certain way. All the dwarf wanted was to be loved, but nothing came as close to the dwarf's face "as big dogs did." And dogs don't have what the dwarf needs. I could hardly breathe.

The next poem was by the same guy. The "volunteers" described a panther, constantly pacing the perimeter of its cage, paralyzed by the bars. No point even trying to breathe. When the students were finished, the strange doctor-who-wants-to-be-my-friend thanked them and the students behind me applauded.

The students then watched part of a film about a man in Victorian England, named Joseph Merrick, who had these huge lumps on his body. He had to hide his appearance to avoid being tormented. The film was called *The Elephant Man*. After the film, the strange doctor-who-wants-to-be-my-friend asked the students to place themselves in the position of Joseph Merrick, the man being tormented because of his appearance. He asked them "What is it that Joseph Merrick wanted in life?"

The students responded with words like "equality," "understanding," "dignity," and "love." It really is too bad these students have to grow up to become doctors.

The strange doctor then tells his students that they have a "professional obligation" to advocate not only for their patients, like the physician in the movie does for Joseph Merrick, but also to advocate for the health of everyone in their community, to promote both their physical and emotional well-being. He tells them they must particularly advocate for those not able to advocate for themselves. I'll have to be careful of this guy and keep reminding myself that he's still a doctor.

Chapter 11

May 6, 2000

When I walked to the door of the meeting room
I was greeted by a woman
Whose voice was not that of the woman on the phone
But who knew my name.
She asked if I could share a few words about Ruth.
I looked down and shook my head.
"Only if you want to."
I shook my head again.
"Only when you're ready to."
How can I be "ready to"
Reeking of remorse about her life
Self-recrimination about her death.
I started to speak but stopped.
Instead I walked to a chair at the edge of a row
That seemed slightly apart from the others
Sat down and looked at the floor.

All Friends sit silently
Patiently
Waiting
Waiting.

Chapter 12

November 16, 1997

The group home's newest attendant just left my room after performing my morning ablutions as instructed to last week by another attendant who's been here a few months more. Like all new attendants, this one's very careful and deliberate and very nervous around me, even though she tries to smile constantly, which I appreciate though, of course, I never could admit that something like smiling helps.

She's fresh from completing the six-week course on how to care for people who can't get their asses in gear by themselves. She must be very bright because in just six short weeks, she learned to look after old people, paraplegic people, post-stroke people, not to mention us quads. She learned to bathe us, feed us, brush our teeth, and change our diapers. She learned to change our urine bags without flooding the floor, and learned to turn us so we won't get bedsores. She must have had very bright teachers who know so much, and can teach so much in six weeks.

The owners of these new training schools must also be very bright if they can hire teachers who can teach these students to learn so much in six weeks, so much so that they qualify for our health system. It's amazing how much they have to learn and have to remember to take good care of us. I bet neither the caregiver training companies nor any of their instructors mention to their students that they won't have time to do what they are being taught to do because there will be far too many of us care-ees to take care of, for each of them lucky enough to be hired by some company. Or at least I'm sure they don't mention this until after tuition is collected in full.

I like this new kid. Still enthusiastic. Still smiling all the time after her first week. Hasn't been exhausted by the work yet. Hasn't complained about the short staff yet. Not even grumbled. Likely because all the attendants really appreciate having a job, even a minimum-wage job, especially at first. But once they're sure that no more caregivers will ever be hired to help them, they sort of give up. Many don't last more than a few months. I hope this one will.

Chapter 13

January 30, 1999

It's really cold and snowy out there.

Do you know that Victoria, British Columbia, is the most wheelchair-friendly city in Canada? First of all, it doesn't snow in Victoria. Snow and ice and salt are, of course, tough on wheelchairs, even power chairs like mine, and tougher on those who use them.

Second, all the sidewalks in Victoria have wheelchair ramps. I mean *all* the sidewalks. I'm most interested in the sidewalks that lead down to the beautiful bay in the centre of the city, where the float planes land and take off, usually from and to Vancouver. I also like the trail along the ocean, "breathtaking views," and lots of friendly dogs with reasonably responsible owners.

Third, apparently the city is full of the extra-large electric doors that truly are wheelchair-accessible, and not just the electronic "press-to-open" discs that are of no use to me, and, I understand, rarely work anyway, but they have light-sensitive electronic door openers that, believe it or not, always work. Fourth, Victoria has large wheelchair-friendly elevators, not only in public buildings but in theatres and malls. For some of the elevators, you can actually call out your floor number and the elevator repeats it, and then tells you when you've arrived on that floor.

I personally know a lot about Victoria because I hitchhiked out there with a girlfriend when I was seventeen. We waitressed all summer. It was a cool place to be. I know a lot about its wheelchair accessibility from speaking with other people with disabilities who have computers and can actually turn them on and look things up on the Net. Apparently Victoria has the highest concentration of both hippies and people who need a little assistance, like older people and people "like me." So now that the two have come together, I hope to move to Victoria soon. Move there before they decide to let me die here. But, I hear it's an expensive place to live. So I'll have to find the do-re-mi.

Chapter 14

April 27, 1998

This Monday Night, he runs into the hospital's amphitheatre with a whole three minutes to spare. Of course, I am sitting in the same place, as they have not made it more wheelchair-friendly in the past two months. Of course, he gives me the same stunned look, then a sympathetic look, and says, "I'm sorry you're back in hospital, Ruth."

"Actually I'm not back in hospital, Doc."

"You're not?"

"Open your eyes, Doc. Am I wearing my elegant hospital gown?"

"Well how —"

"A van moves us disableds out of our storage facilities and back in again. It brought me tonight."

He's not sure he believes me. Maybe he got hit by part of the shit storm that occurred after I illegally came to his compassion session last time. He looks me up and down, trying to assure himself that my being in street clothes, really means I'm not an "in patient" and therefore am allowed here. He says, "I'm glad you're not ill again, Ruth." Then he smiles and says, "In fact, you're looking very well tonight."

Give me a break. What does he want now? But there's no time to ask him because he quickly runs away to the centre of the amphitheatre and welcomes the students before I can throw him off again. He finishes his welcome with, "Students, our friend, Ruth, has joined us again this evening, let's welcome her," as if they were in nursery school, or on *Mister Rogers' Neighborhood*.

I hear them clapping behind me. I debate pirouetting my chair to take an acknowledging bow, but as neither my body nor chair bow to anybody, I decide to pretend I don't hear them.

This Monday Night's not as powerful. Just one very long one-woman Victorian-type play about mental illness. The doc-who-wants-to-be-my-friend told the students he adapted it from a short story — with "permission of the estate of the author" no less. I do like the way the play shows how a woman can be confined by the times in which she lives — and by the medical profession. It really is going on too long though. My piss bag is going to burst. The doc-who-wants-to-be-my-friend will have to learn how to get to the point quicker if he wants this stuff to work.

At about the three-hour mark, the medical student–actor actually has me convinced that she has gradually gone insane. Probably from all the lines she has been reciting. I realize that she has memorized all these lines. I don't think she's needed prompting for any of the thousands and thousands of lines. You know, I bet she'll remember every line of every medical textbook she ever reads. She also seems very sensitive. I definitely want her to be my doctor, on both counts.

When the "exploration" is over, a bunch of students surround me. They ask me how I am feeling, how I liked the play, what I thought about the woman being confined like that, and a bunch of other questions before I can respond to the first. I can only see the students directly in front of me, but all of them are women. I tell them I was very impressed with their buddy who had to memorize all the lines. Cruel and unusual punishment — both the character's confinement and the actor having to memorize all those lines.

Out of the corner of my left eye, I see my strange doctor-friend, with a grin stretched across his face. He looks like the

Cheshire Cat in Disney's *Alice in Wonderland*, except that he's wearing a black jacket and black turtleneck sweater. He wore that same outfit last time. Must be his Monday Night teaching costume. He'd look better in Cheshire Cat stripes.

After all the students are gone, he walks over, still grinning, and asks if he can "accompany" me to the van. I pivot my chair and rapidly head out the amphitheatre doors. He catches up, but stupidly walks behind my chair as if he is pushing it. He's talking to me as if he thinks I can turn my head at any time to acknowledge his stupid conversation-making. What a dolt.

When we come to the large closed doors that separate the lecture halls from the rest of the hospital, he dashes round my chair, pretends to sweep off a Three Musketeers' hat, as he bows like a cavalier before opening the damn doors for me. So ridiculous.

I power off. He catches up, still trying to make small talk, telling me my "chair sounds like a vacuum cleaner, no, a golf cart."

I say, "I assume you play golf, like all doctors."

I think that offended him for some reason, but I can't really tell because he's still behind me, pretending to push my chair. Finally he comes out with,

"I'm sorry to disappoint you but I'm afraid I don't have the time."

A touch of sarcasm perhaps. There's hope for him then. So of course I ask,

"Then how do you know what a golf cart sounds like?"

That was a mistake because he starts prattling on about how when his father came to visit him in California when he was on a cancer research fellowship there, he took his Dad to this famous golf course above the ocean that was on TV all the time. It overlooked the ocean, and he knew his father would love to play there. But the golf course had a rule that you had to use a golf cart, and renting the cart cost an outrageous amount of money, more than the fee to play. He said his father was physically fit in those days, and they felt more cheated not being able to walk on the bluffs above the sea than by the outrageous cash grab. Why is he telling me this story?

I speed down the hall to the elevators. He chases after me, but I'm too fast for him, of course. So I get to the elevators first and patiently wait. He eventually arrives, puffing, blushing, apologizing. After he catches his breath, he just stands there smiling at me, Cheshire Cat again. I just stare straight ahead at the puke-green elevator doors.

When I can't stand his grinning-down-my-neck any longer, I say, "I noticed you're adequate at opening doors, let's see if you can press the elevator button." He's slow on the uptake and doesn't move.

"The one with the arrow pointing down please."

He steps forward presses the down button, cranks his lowered face around to mine, and gives me a looking-for-approval smile. Sure. I nod my eyebrows. His smile broadens. So proud of himself.

The elevator comes quickly as "Visitors' hours are now over." The doors open. He offers a deep Elizabethan bow, and extends his left arm against the left elevator door to protect me from it closing on me, which, even though I'm lightning with this chair, happens quite frequently, but he doesn't need to know about that. I quickly pirouette my chair, but instead of backing in as fast as I can, as I usually do, so the doors won't hit my chair and open again, I back in very slowly. I hear the elevator doors closing and opening against his left arm over and over again, and his embarrassed voice saying, "Sorry, sorry, sorry" over and over again. I bet he's not smiling now. He wants to feel useful after all. And I want him to feel useful after all, so let him fend off the offending doors that now start to beep.

He says, "Sorry, sorry" to the beeping as well, even more embarrassed, and I mercifully accelerate my completion of entering the elevator, even though I know that when the beeping starts, the doors will stay open a few seconds and then slowly close.

He calmly tells me how amazed he is by my "dexterity" with my chair and compliments me with, "You're quite skilled at this."

"Years of practice," I murmur. "And it's chinexterity if you look closely."

He smiles, trying to think of something clever enough to say to keep up with my wit, but of course he cannot.

The elevator doors finally begin to close again, and he quickly jumps in, but not quickly enough, and the doors close on both his shoulders, which of course triggers the doors to open again. He's embarrassed but still grinning as the doors finally shut. However, his smile disappears when the elevator goes up because Doc here stood there grinning at me instead of pressing "G" to send it down.

Again embarrassed, he says, "I'm sorry," and quickly presses "G," telling me, "Someone must have pressed an elevator button on a floor above us so the elevator has to go up before I can turn it around."

"No kidding, Doc."

Then he starts rapidly firing off that he has claustrophobia, has had "claustrophobia since age fifteen because of a recurring dream," and then a bunch of other nervous gibberish I can't make out, and don't care a hoot about, until the doors finally open on the tenth floor. He jumps out, a nurse gets in, smiles at me, looks at him, probably like he's weird but I can't see her face now, and then she presses "5." He jumps in, but too late and the doors close on him. They open again, they close, and the elevator finally goes down.

The doors open on the fifth floor, and the nurse says, "Good night" as she gets off.

I think Doc is embarrassed and staring at his feet, looking a little green, although all that's hard to tell, as I am staring straight ahead. Then I see him quickly dashing forward to press "G."

"Good boy," I say encouragingly.

The elevator descends and lands on the ground floor. Doc exhales when the doors open and bolts out, almost tripping because the elevator floor is a little lower than "ground floor," a fact that those of us in chairs have known for some time. He then dashes back into the elevator to help my chair over the bump. But of course no one needs to help my power chair climb over a little elevator bump. I'll put my power chair up against any ATV. So before his hands reach my chair's non-existent handles, I jut my chin forward and blast out of the door before he can pretend to think that he's helping me.

I beeline for the front doors, even though I know the automatic doors don't work after nine because "Visitors' hours are now over," and the hospital has this security thing. It's after nine, of course, because the strange doctor-who-wants-to-be-my-friend doesn't know how to put on a short play, or how to push "G" when getting on an elevator. I stop at the front doors and stare outside. He catches up, panting and smiling.

I tell him, "I would like to wait outside. It's a beautiful evening after all."

He proudly presses the ALARM WILL SOUND lever-bar on the hospital door, at the same time proudly soothing me with,

"Don't worry, the alarm won't sound, I always use this door at night to get to my car faster."

Such a rebel. He'd be disappointed to know that I wasn't worried in the slightest about the door's alarm sounding. I have exited through these doors after "Visitors' hours are now over" many times over the years. I just have to wait patiently for someone on staff like him, who also knows the deep dark secret that the alarm won't sound, to press the bar for me on their way out to their car.

Even if the alarm *did* sound, no one would worry as alarms are going off around here all the time. On the contrary, even when the voice calmly says "Code Red" and the location, meaning there's a fire at that location, no one reacts because everyone assumes it's a mock fire drill, or someone has pulled the fire alarm inadvertently; and of course the woman, whose calm voice we hear, either knows that there's no real fire, or doesn't know but is told to use her calmest voice in all circumstances, which I can dig. Same thing for "Code White" and "Code Yellow" and "Code Chartreuse." It's only when her voice comes over the PA calmly saying "Code Blue" and the location, which means someone's heart has stopped at that location, that people actually react. Then you see "crash carts" flying with staff trying to catch up to them.

Chapter 15

April 27, 1998

I quickly dash out the door into what's left of the beautiful evening, turn sharply left without losing speed, and motor toward the sign that reads "Smoking is prohibited within 9 metres of the hospital's entrance" (which we smokers all intentionally interpret as nine feet, an improvement over the previous thirty feet until we got tired of security guards explaining to us what a "metre" was). I turn my chair and stop a few feet before the sign, as I always do, leaving skid marks, as I always do.

He catches up, panting, and squeezes out, "May I have your permission to wait with you?"

The "permission" thing again. What a nutbag.

I tell him, "The van's usually late. Actually it's already late as I had no idea your play would be so incredibly long."

He looks hurt, poor boy.

"It may still not be here for an hour or more."

"I'd really like to wait with you," he sheepishly says.

I assure him, "I'm a big girl," and tell him to "Go home."

His feet stay planted. He just stares at me.

"I would still like to wait with you if that's okay," he quietly pleads.

I just stare at him. Then I tell him "The van may have already come, and because I was not out here patiently waiting because of the turtle pace of your play, probably took off somewhere. I wouldn't be surprised if the van has already come back and left again and probably forgot about me by now."

This takes a while to sink into his thick head and he slumps his shoulders. But then he perks up again because he really doesn't believe me. He should. But he thinks I'm teasing him, which of course I would never do.

Finally, he smiles and says, "I really would like to wait with you. 'It's a beautiful evening after all.'" And extends his smile to Cheshire Cat length.

Touché, he thinks.

"Okay, Doc, you can wait with me but only if you make yourself useful. Fetch me a cig from the sack hanging behind my chair." He's not smiling now. Just the opposite.

"You smoke?" he whispers.

"Of course not, smoking would be bad for my health."

He tries not to glance at the NO SMOKING sign behind my right shoulder, but keeps glancing at it anyway, surreptitiously, he thinks. I don't tell him that I always smoke here just before the sign, just to see if any security guard has the rocks to make me move beyond the nine-metre mark. None of them ever ask me to move. In fact, they pretend not to see me smoking here, and avoid eye contact as their feet give me a wide berth as they walk past me. The security guards are all afraid of me for some reason. I've often wondered how these big guys can be afraid of a sweet little woman like me. A sweet defenceless woman who's less than half their size and can't even walk, let alone lift my arm, clench my fist, and throw a punch. Maybe they think what I have is contagious, and that they might catch it from me. Nah. Even doctors, who must know that I'm not contagious, are still afraid of me for some reason.

He's still staring at me, trying not to see the NO SMOKING sign.

"Ahem, my cigs, please."

He raises his eyebrows, and gives me an I'm-not-so-sure-about-this look. "C'mon, Doc, snap to it."

He walks around to the back of my chair. I can't see him, but he's probably staring at my bag. I can understand why he's staring at my bag. It's a lovely bag, left over from my hippy days. It's made of woven wool in many earth tones and is fringed with knotted strands of rainbow colours, of course with painted wooden beads sprinkled here and there. Maybe he's having a warm nostalgic moment about a girl he knew who carried a bag like this. So many of us did. Nah, he was probably too busy with medical school to go out with girls.

Finally I hear one of his hands start gingerly feeling around in there. He's probably embarrassed to have his hand in a woman's purse, afraid of what he might touch. Probably thinks it's bad manners. His mother taught him well. He's probably fumbling his way around my wallet and life's essentials. Then with a *voilà*, he pulls out my pack of *Luckies* and holds it in front of my face — and holds it front of my face — and holds it in front of my face. I'm always amazed at what they let into medical school.

I'm having a nicotine fit here and he keeps on holding my pack of *Luckies* like he's posing for a billboard ad. But of course he doesn't have any idea what he's doing, and he's not nearly macho enough to pull it off anyway. If I could just get my hands around his fucking throat. But as I'm a lady, I clench my jaws tight to keep "stupid turd" in my throat. Then I very politely in my best Maggie Smith *Miss Jean Brodie* say,

"Now please take a cigarette out of the pack, my dear boy."

He hesitates, then slowly draws a *Lucky* out of the pack as if it's a nuclear rod. Then he holds the *Lucky* vertically, as far away from both him and me as possible without moving his feet — and holds it — and holds it.

"Now into my mouth please."

He doesn't move a muscle. No sign of life except his eyes are open, and he's standing of course.

"I promise not to tell anyone that you're hastening my death."

He blushes but remains frozen. He's a blushing iceberg, and I'm getting really pissed off. You'd be pissed off too if a cig was taunting you mere inches from your mouth.

"Just put the fucking thing in my mouth!"

He shoves the cigarette so deep into my mouth that I'm gagging.

I garble, "Take it out, you dimwit."

He leans over and puts his ear closer to my mouth because he couldn't make out what I said. I knew I would probably choke to death one day, but please, not like this.

"Take it out, stupid."

He finally gets what I'm saying and pulls the cigarette out, saying, "Sorry, sorry, sorry," over and over as if it's the end of the world. It would be the end of his world if I could get my hands on his throat. I'd show him what choking feels like.

I regain my composure, but only barely, and only because I need my nicotine, but I can't do a proper lady anymore.

"Put the fucking cigarette back in."

He starts to.

"Stop. Just a little way in this time."

He very gently places the cigarette at the edge of my lips. It's going to fall out, so I tightly clamp on to it with my lip tips, and try to suck it in with all the suck I have left. Then I rotate my lips with all I have to move it further into my mouth.

"In okay?" he stupidly asks.

"Would I be working my mouth like a camel if it's in okay?" I'm not sure he understands what I'm saying because I'm mumbling as if I have marbles in my mouth so the cigarette won't fall out.

But he gets the drift, says, "I'm sorry" again and gently pushes the cigarette in further.

"Okay stop."

I take a deep breath, glad that that's over with. He just stands there, stupidly staring at my cigarette as if it's hypnotizing him.

I just sit here patiently waiting, staring at his stupid face, until I can't take it any longer.

"You fucking don't expect me just to suck on this thing as if it's a fucking candy cigarette."

That untrances him, and he starts again with, "I'm sorry," over and over again until he finally asks, "Do you have any matches in your purse?"

I almost say, "Dah, what do you think you fucking asshole?" but because I'm a lady, I just glare.

Eventually he gets the message and cautiously begins excavating my bag again. I'm dying here. It seems to be taking longer than last time. I guess the match folder is harder to find than my pack of *Luckies*.

He finally comes up with the matches, so proud of himself, holds them in front of my face, like he did with my pack of *Luckies*. Realizes what he's doing again, so this time he quickly bows and asks, "Do you want me to light your cigarette for you?" as if he's a maître d' in a fancy restaurant in the movies.

I'm ready to kill him, but go with it in my best Billy Crystal's Fernando Lamas voice, "That would be M-A-H-V-E-L-O-U-S, thank you," and add, "That is, if you think you can light it without burning my face." But I immediately worry the joke will be on me.

He struggles with the matches like he's never lit one before. He scratches and scratches. And scratches and scratches. Finally a flame, but it goes out before it reaches my cig. Probably because his hands are shaking like he has a neurological condition himself. I'm glad he's never going to operate on me.

I wish I could steady his hands in mine like Barbara Stanwyck does in the movies. The next match gets to my *Lucky*, and I start frantically puffing for my life. The flame goes out anyway. More scratching. Then a flame. Then up to my cig again. More puffing, and Ahh…Ahh.

I cradle the cig in the corner of my mouth. He stares at me for a bit, then he says, "You look like a movie gangster with the cigarette in the corner of your mouth like that."

I ignore him.

Then he says, "Tell me everything, you understand, everything," in a poor attempt at an Edward G. Robinson voice. You know, I'm not sure if he's trying to make a movie gangster joke, or whether it's the line from the Spielberg kids' movie, *Goonies*, where a kid, instead of telling the gangsters "everything" about the buried treasure, tells the gangsters "everything" about himself. I assume the strange doctor has kids. I think most doctors have kids. So I go with it, but instead of telling the strange doctor with the strange gangster voice "everything" he wants to know about me, I tell him "everything" he doesn't want to know about his healthcare system.

I love how he flinches in pain each time I skewer his profession, which he apparently loves, and definitely has endless excuses for, like: "We've less than half the doctors per citizen of any developed country," and "We do the best we can considering the cuts to hospital funding," and "Canada now has half the doctors per population of any developed country because of the cutbacks to medical school positions."

I tell him, "That doesn't sound very developed to me." I keep to myself that if a doctor who teaches what he does, and believes what he just said, and does nothing to change the system but just makes excuses for it, we're screwed. You are what you do, not what you say, asshole.

He goes on pontificating about something, oblivious to the fact that I'm totally focused on enjoying my cig. After a while I hear, "In addition, the number of nurses per patient has been slashed, as has the extent of the training of the caregivers who are replacing them."

He's got me listening a bit now.

"All because of the slash of health funding since the last election to fulfill the campaign promise of personal income tax breaks."

He has my full attention, but he's slowing down. He starts talking so slowly that I think he's having trouble finding his words, like some people who have had a stroke. I realize he's distracted by trying not to stare at the bobbing ash of my cig, particularly when some falls on my shawl. I know he wants to brush the ash off my shawl, but is afraid to touch me. Finally he stops mid-sentence and timidly brushes the air above the shawl. When he's sure I'm not going to ignite, he cautiously starts revving up his rant.

"Cutbacks in personal income taxes hurt rather than benefit the people who need health promotion and care most. They don't have the money to get around the system, like going to the States, or having a connection that could jump a waiting list. So don't blame physicians, blame the politicians and the citizens who voted them in." He stops cold, worrying my cig's getting too short, and my lips will burn. He steps off his soapbox and asks, "Can I take it out?"

"Sure if it's making you nervous, but you're wasting good tobacco."

He gently removes the butt from my lips, and looks for a place to dump it. He starts walking farther away from the hospital's door. I turn my chair to watch him. He's holding the butt as far away from his body as possible, like it's a lit firecracker. After about twenty feet, he finds a metal trash cylinder that has a sand-filled ashtray on stilts above its opening. After dropping my cig on the sand, he tentatively pokes at it with his finger. Then takes a good look to make sure it's out. He turns and slowly walks back to me. He looks stressed out. Good.

"Light me another, thank-you-very-much."

He sighs, but walks around my chair anyway, and begins searching my purse again. Of course my *Luckies* are no longer in my purse. He dropped them on the ground when he realized I was strangling on my cig. I patiently wait. When it hits him where my pack of *Luckies* must be, he blushes and nonchalantly picks up the pack, hoping I didn't notice.

This time, still struggling, he gently places the cig at the appropriate depth in my mouth, then lights a match with his still shaking hands. But he is able to bring the flame to my cig in time for me to take a good drag. I'm feeling much better now. Even in a generous mood. So I ask him,

"Hey, Doc, you wanna cig?"

He says, "No thank you," and becomes a docsicle again.

"What's wrong? You don't like *Luckies*, eh? Well you sure don't look like a 'Marlboro Man' to me, so why not give a *Lucky* a try?"

He stays there frozen until I ask him for another cigarette.

I usually have just one cig in the evening, but it's such a riot watching a doctor struggle for a change, that I keep asking him to light me cig after cig. He tries not to look relieved when the van arrives. I try not to look disappointed. I was hoping the driver forgot about me. That happens, you know.

Tonight's driver, a burly guy about our age, walks around to our side of the van. He smiles as he swings open the barn doors and presses the button that lowers the elevator platform. I gun my chair forward onto the platform, "Thanks for the drags, Doc," and am hauled up and into the van.

As there is no room in the van to turn my chair, I stare out the window on the opposite side at a vacant bus shelter under a yellowish streetlight. I hear the ratcheting down of my chair to the van's floor, then the metallic thud of the closed doors. The driver walks across my view. His weight enters the van. The motor rumbles on. The bus shelter and streetlight move left and are gone.

Suddenly I see my strange doctor-friend. He's running beside the window, frantically waving goodbye with both hands, and mouthing like an orangutan, "T-H-A-N-K — Y-O-U — F-O-R — C-O-M-I-N-G." He's going to get hit by a car.

Now I think he's saying, "C-A-L-L — M-E — I-F — T-H-E-R-E'S — A-N-Y-T-H-I-N-G — I — C-A-N — D-O — F-O-R — Y-O-U."

Then he stops mouthing, but keeps running beside the window, still waving both hands. Finally he disappears left. Probably collapsed on the street.

Chapter 16

May 6, 2000

A long while passes.
The voice of the woman who met me at the door
Says, "Our friend Ruth
Always in good humour.
Her wonderful wit
Probably went over my head often as not.
It was hard to tell
Because her eyes always had that wry smile.
She was always uplifting."

I lift my eyes.
The woman seems to be looking straight at me.
I look away,
Scanning the other women
Contemplation mixes with smiles around me.

Another woman begins speaking.
She talks about Ruth's barbed questions
That she had to consider carefully
Before daring to answer.
She worried that even acknowledging the question
Let alone answering the question
Was the intended end of Ruth's humour.
Her smile broadened.

She finishes too soon for me.
The ensuing silence consumes me.

Chapter 17

September 28, 1998

I'm back in hospital. Nothing serious this time, just some plumbing problems.

I saw that strange doctor-supposed-friend today while I was bombing down the halls on his floor. He was about to enter the stairwell. Unfortunately, he saw me, too, while I was still accelerating, and he had time to duck into the stairwell at the last second, or I would have flattened him good.

With all his "I want to be friends" bullshit, he never visited me at the group home. Not even once. And the group home is so close to the hospital. Some friend. You know, I don't think we've talked more than half a dozen times in total. And two have been when I came to his Monday Night compassion sessions. It's not easy for me to call him, let alone arrange to meet up with him at Timmie's.

Anyway, after he peeks out of the stairwell and sees me motoring away, he chases after me down the hallway as if I had stolen his wallet, except that he's yelling, "Stop, Ruth," instead of "Stop, thief." I decide to let him catch up. When he does, I give him, in an even snootier *Miss Jean Brodie*, "Is there anything I can do for you?"

When he finally catches his breath, he sort of barks like a seal, "Are you ill again?"

"Me, ill? Of course not."

He breathes a couple more times and asks, "Why are you back in hospital?"

Still in Maggie Smith, I tell him, "It's nothing for you to be concerned about, my dear boy."

He asks my room number so he can visit me later. I am hesitant to give it to him, but I do, knowing that as he knows my name and he's a doctor, he could find my room number if he wanted to anyway, that is if he took the time to find out. He thanks me and dashes off down the hall, and back into the stairwell.

You know, when we talk, albeit always briefly, he seems to care so much about me, but if he cared about me, he would have visited me at the group home. I have to almost crash into him, or park my chair in front of his precious medical students, before he remembers I exist.

Chapter 18

September 28, 1998

I bumped into Ruth today. She's back in hospital. Looks okay though. Actually Ruth almost bumped into me. She lost control of her wheelchair when she was hurrying over to say hello, and really came close to crashing into me.

I told her how glad I was to see her, but she misunderstood and said, "You're glad I'm back in this ___ place?"

She used an adjective before "place" because she doesn't like hospitals.

I was late for a meeting and did not have time to talk with her. I will try to see her after work.

Chapter 19

September 28, 1998

I wasn't always a patient woman. Far from it. I think I've been impatient since I was a little kid. By the time I got to high school I impatiently couldn't wait to get out of high school and its rules, like no smoking on the school grounds, which of course resulted in the neighbouring properties being littered by butts and other detritus associated with a herd of high-schoolers standing on your lawn: matches, Kleenex, post-cig bubble gum wrappers. Rules like wearing long skirts, at least long enough to touch the ground if you were told to drop to your knees, which teachers, of course, had us do if they thought our skirts were sinfully short, which they always were because girls were not allowed to wear pants, and it was the sixties after all. So we of course had to install clips to surreptitiously hook the hem back up until the next teacher saw you in the hall and asked you to drop to your knees, again to check your skirt. Obviously it was the female teachers that had you drop to your knees. The male teachers didn't seem to mind short skirts. The boys also seemed to like short skirts, especially when sitting across the circle from a girl in Senior English, where a trying-to-be-avant-garde male teacher had the desks organized in a circle. It was ironic that it was in English class that the boys lost any ability they had to speak English, not that they could comment on Shakespeare in French or any other language even if we sat in straight rows and wore pants. Garbling the English language was probably an accompanying symptom of the sinful sunburn they always seemed to have in English class.

I impatiently couldn't wait to get out of my parents' house and its rules, like no smoking, like play your radio quiet so only you can hear it, like having to put on your lipstick after you leave the house. Blame it on rock and roll, not me, momma.

In art school, I was impatient with drawing. Very impatient. For that matter, I was even impatient with waiting my turn at the kiln, sometimes for days, to see what my glazes would eventually bake on my clay. Then, in my artist days I would impatiently pace back and forth across my studio while waiting to see what Fred, taking his fine sweet time, would create with our enamel pieces on our carved copper. I smoked cig after cig while waiting for Fred.

So when I got sick, and learned why patients are called patients, I had no choice but to learn to be a patient patient. Most of us patients are in the same boat because there are too many patients booked to see doctors at the exact same time. Too many patients, not enough doctors, not enough time. So I've learned to be a patient patient, or at least learned to pretend to be a patient patient. Wouldn't want to seem impolite or unappreciative. The doctors, nurses, and receptionists think it's easier for me to be a patient patient than most. They think people "like me" after all have nowhere to rush off to, nowhere important to be. They assume I have no children to pick up, no exciting things waiting for me that patiently waiting keeps me from doing.

Family members also have to learn to be patient while the overbooked doctor is cramming through his "list." And family members don't get a dime for waiting-room time, or transportation time, or help-at-home time. They even have to pay out of pocket to park in the hospital lot. I have heard some argue that keeping us kept waiting for hours is a purposeful program the hospital initiated following the "cutbacks," and that it actually did work to help the hospital balance its budget. It's harder for family members to be patient. They have other places to be, other things to do. And patients feel guilty because their family members are being kept waiting.

Most of the time, it is really hard for me to be a patient patient. I feel like charging my power chair through the receptionist's barricade, right through the clinic doors, past the nurses, and straight into the doctor. Hit him in the knees so he can't help but see me when he bends over in pain. I have a better chance of nailing a doctor when the clinic is in the hospital, because they sometimes have to be brave enough to leave the clinic area through the waiting room — I guess to go to Emerg, or to see a patient on the ward, or go to a meeting.

When I see a doctor who was supposed to see me an hour or more ago head out of the clinic, I always head toward him, trying to catch his eye. The doctor always averts his eyes, pretending not to see me. Sometimes a doctor will give me a quick acknowledging glance before he quickly turns his head away so I cannot suck onto his eyes more firmly. A "Hello" and an "I'm sorry I'm running late" is all that would be required for me to be a patient patient. But that would slow them down for a second or two, and seconds or twos add up, and put them farther behind, which of course irritates them when they know they're already running way late. Overall, though, for almost twenty-seven years now, I think I have been a patient patient.

But I am "No Longer Patient." As a matter of fact, I am the most impatient patient who ever existed. I need my joystick connected to my computer. Now. I have waited almost three years and cannot wait any longer. There are things I want to learn, places I want to see, words I need to write. And no doctor thought I would live this long.

Chapter 20

May 6, 2000

A long while passes.
Friends privately celebrate Ruth's life.
Silence surrounds me.
Finally another woman begins to speak.
She tells another story about "our Friend's great sense of humour."
All are warmly and tearfully smiling
Except me.

She finishes too soon for me.

More silence.
Another woman says
"Ruth knew a lot about old movies."
Heads nod.
All smile
Except me.

Chapter 21

September 28, 1998

He rushes into my room, with his usual greeting, caring, concern-for-my-health bullshit, but he's already got one foot out the door, like all doctors. He doesn't even take the time today to draw the curtain around my bed. How long does it take to whip a curtain along its ceiling rod for ten feet?

After a few minutes of his looking intensely interested in me like he always seems to, pretending not to be in a hurry to leave, he looks down at his feet. This is what he always does just before he starts apologizing for having to leave. He will soon ask me if there's anything I need like he always does just before he leaves. I will just stare at him like I always do when he's getting ready to leave. But this time he changes things up with,

"Since you're back in hospital and looking so well …"

I of course know something's coming. He probably wants to display me in front of his students. So I throw him off with,

"No you can't show my VULVA to your students."

That threw him off, all right. I haven't seen him frozen solid with his mouth open for a while. When he shakes his head to recover, I stop him again with,

"You can't show my VULVA to any of your students."

"No …"

"Not even a female student."

He just stares for a while with his mouth open. I'm happy to make him late for something.

He finally starts up again with, "No, no, no, you don't understand. This has nothing to do with my students. I just wanted to ask your permission to bring my children in to meet you."

Well, well, well. And he hasn't surprised me for a while either.

"Permission ... children ... "

He pushes onward quickly before I throw him off again.

"It would only be for a few minutes, and only if you're feeling well enough to, and only if you want to."

He sheepishly stares at me. I glare back.

He whispers, "Please feel free to say no, if you'd rather not."

Permission to bring in his kids, give me a break. Does this nutbar think I could possibly say, "No, I don't want to meet your kids?" So of course I say, "I would like to meet your kids."

I realize he has been actually holding his breath waiting because he exhales a big sigh of relief. He says, "Thank you, I will bring them to your room in about an hour and a half."

He turns and starts to leave, but of course I'm not going to make it that easy for him. "Not in my room. We don't want to disturb the other patients. Let's all meet in my favourite part of the hospital instead."

He starts to speak but stops. He looks at his feet then hesitantly pretends to inquire, "Favourite part?"

"Yes, favourite part. You know exactly where."

He's still looking at his feet, pretending not to know that he knows exactly where I mean to meet up. He's also pretending not to believe I would do this to him, but in fact knowing I would definitely do this to him. Then he even more hesitantly says,

"I'm not sure I know ..."

"Of course you do."

And then, he whispers, "Where?" with such sweet innocence.

"Outside the front doors."

"Well, I don't ... ah ..."

"It's a beautiful evening after all." Gotcha.

He hesitates, then stammers, "I'm not sure that location is such a good idea."

I just stare at him.

He's still staring down at his feet. He begins to shift his weight from one foot to the other. I'm sure the silence will get to him first, but it doesn't.

"Okay, I promise not to smoke in front of your kids."

He exhales, "Thank you" and rushes for the door. But I'm not through with him yet.

"But only if you tell me about your recurring dream."

He stops mid-stride, and looks over his left shoulder at me.

"Recurring dream ...?" he murmurs, as if he has no idea of what I'm referring to.

"You know, the one that makes you claustrophobic in elevators."

"I can't tell you about that," he says quickly and definitively.

"Then I might just ask you in front of your kids if you would join me in another cigarette. *Luckies* are your favourite, aren't they, macho man?"

He's frozen again.

"C'mon, Doc, it's only fair."

"My dream is personal."

"C'mon Doc. You've read my chart and looked at my VULVA and now I want to know just one little personal thing about you and you deny me."

He starts to speak but stops. Then he says,

"Please, I'd rather not talk about my dream. I'll tell you something else that's personal instead."

"It's nonnegotiable. I want the dream. Maybe I can help you get over your claustrophobia."

"I can't."

"I bet you don't want to tell me your dream because you think I'll find you ridiculous?"

"Yes."

"No worries, I already find you ridiculous."

He starts to speak but stops.

"Put your ass on that chair, pretend it's a couch, and tell me your dream."

His scrawny ass abruptly hits the chair and he slowly begins.

"There's a tumultuous lake."

"Very original."

He blushes, looks down at his shoes, "See what I mean."

I actually feel sorry for him, and, believe it or not, I want to apologize, but can't quite do it. So I yawn. I try again to apologize, but, instead, yawn again.

After a while I groan.

"Okay, I promise not to interrupt you again."

He starts speaking, still looking at his shoes, "We are standing on a pier."

"We?"

"The neighbours on the block where I grew up. I'm about fourteen years old. I stand between my mother and Mrs. Warner, the beautiful woman who lives next door. Mrs. Warner is holding the hand of her five-year-old son, Jamie. Jamie was much younger than the rest of us kids. Sort of tagged after us like a puppy. Suddenly a hard wave smashes into the pier and sweeps Jamie into the roiling water."

Yes, he actually says *roiling*.

"Jamie's eyes meet mine just before he is sucked down. My mother grasps my arm and turns me toward her. Her eyes beseech, *Don't*. I love my mother very much, but she knows I'm the strongest swimmer on the street. I dive in confidently, knowing I will rescue Jamie, knowing everyone will be proud of me. However, I can't find Jamie. I duck dive down again, no Jamie. On my fourth dive, I see a cave under the pier and swim into it. I have to swim in quite a way before I finally find Jamie. He's very frightened. I mouth, *Everything will be okay*, grasp his hand, and turn to swim him out. But I see three tunnels. I choose the one in the middle and swim Jamie down it, but it gets narrower and narrower. This can't be the right one. There's hardly room for us to turn around. I swim us back to where I found Jamie and take the tunnel to the left. I swim hard, pulling Jamie. I feel Jamie's body go limp. I'm running out of breath."

My strange doctor-friend is actually gasping out of breath. He's really into this.

"I drag Jamie with all that I have, fighting panic with every stroke. I run out of breath, and wake up gasping for air, drenched in water."

"You mean sweat."

"What?" he pants, bent over, a hand on each knee.

I let him pant for a while.

"Okay, we're making progress now. Besides elevators what else gives your claustrophobia?"

"Being buried in the sand by my kids," he blurts out between breaths.

"Buried in the sand, eh?"

"Buried in the sand is the worst."

"For me too."

He straightens up, stops gasping, looks at me in horror, and runs out of the room.

Chapter 22

September 28, 1998

I pick up my kids and take them to "Wendy's Pick-up Window." They order grilled chicken with broccoli-cheddar baked potatoes, as trained to. I head back to the Hospital. There is silence in the car except for the sounds of chewing jaws. This lack of talking while chewing is very rare. They are feeling the privilege of not being confined to home with schoolwork on a school night.

I have taken the children with me to the Hospital many times before, usually on weekends, ever since each was old enough to patiently wait with the picture books and puzzles stored in the bottom tub drawer in my desk. They call it their drawer. They seemed to not mind waiting there for me while I made morning rounds before taking them to music lessons or soccer practice. They also sometimes came in with me when I was called in to Emerg to see a patient. They haven't wanted to come to the Hospital with me in recent years. Too old now, I guess. But this trip to the Hospital is special. Not just because it is a school night, but because they know they will be meeting someone important to me.

While my children's jaws pensively chew, my brain unwillingly immerses in *To Kill a Mockingbird*. The part where Atticus Finch, the progressive lawyer in a 1930s American South town, sends his twelve-year-old son, Jem, to read to an unconscious woman. Jem would rather be doing anything during his summer holidays than spend his days in an old house, reading to an old woman who does not even know he is there. Periodically, Jem is sent out of the woman's room by a nurse, but just for a few minutes. Over the weeks of that summer, Jem believes that the woman is becoming more responsive to his reading. He also notices the nurse comes into the room less frequently and finally not at all. When the woman starts acknowledging him, Jem wonders whether she could hear him reading to her all the time. The woman dies a few weeks later, and Atticus explains to his son that she had been taking medicine to control the great pain she was in from the illness that eventually caused her death, but had insisted on backing off the pain medicine so that she could experience life again before she died.

I read the book to my children a few years ago. I also brought home the film version for one of our "Thursday Night at the Movies." I first read *To Kill a Mockingbird* when I was a teenager and have reread it several times since. Atticus Finch was who I wanted to be, but not because of this part of the novel. As a matter of fact, I always read the part of the dying woman quickly because I wanted to get back to Atticus and the civil liberties part, and I don't think the dying woman was even in the movie. So it's not until I am pulling the car into the "Doctors' Parking Lot" I realize for the first time that Atticus sent Jem to read to the old woman so that his son could learn from her. Learn courage from her. But also learn the importance of each hour of life: learn its beauty from her, learn its wonder from her. Even though the woman could not leave her bed or even lift her head.

Chapter 23

September 28, 1998

I catch a friendly nurse who has come into the room to see one of the other inmates. I ask her if she has time to get me into my chair, change my piss bag, and throw my shawl on my shoulders.

She gives me a big smile and says, "No problem, Dearie. I have all the time in the world for you."

She's from Jamaica, but that was years ago, and I think she lays on the accent just to make me smile. I try not to smile back. Can't ruin my image. But it's hard to stop my face stretching and teeth from showing every time this nurse comes into the room. She gently, as well as jokingly complies with my requests, although she pretends to give me a hard time about it. Even calls me a "little princess" sometimes when I'm very precise as to where the TV needs to be and what channel it should be tuned to.

When she has me snug in my chair, she decides to brush my hair, even though she knows I'm itching to hit the halls. She brushes very slowly and gently, and keeps brushing my hair even after I smile and say, "Enough already."

She stops for a moment, pretends to assess her work, and says, "Whose heart you going to break tonight, Dearie?"

A moment is all I need. My chin presses my joystick as far forward as it can, and I hit the halls with time to spare to my favourite spot of the hospital, and, if I'm lucky, get a fellow imbiber to light a *Lucky* for me, place it between my lips, and smoke it before his kids show up.

I'm kind of interested in seeing what his children are like. I'm sure they're interested in seeing what I'm like. That is, if he's told his kids about me, which he probably hasn't. Too busy with important things to talk about with them, and important things to teach them. Like how to kick a soccer ball or play the piano, or whatever. If he hasn't told his kids about me yet, he will any minute now.

He will start with, of course, "I want you to meet my friend, Ruth." Probably in the same serious voice he uses for his medical students. He will then prepare them for what they will see, which of course wasn't possible for his medical students, them seeing me before he rushed into the amphitheatre. But of course medical students have seen patients like me before so they need no preparation.

He'll probably describe me as a very nice woman who drives a very fast little car. Maybe she'll show you how fast it can go. But don't ask her if you can drive it. Maybe he'll tell them she's like Pollyanna after her accident and can't walk anymore, like Hayley Mills in the Disney film. I am very Pollyanna-like as a matter of fact, always optimistic about life, though I, of course, can't show it, as that would be bad for my reputation. He might tell them my language isn't quite as pleasant as Pollyanna's, but I mean nothing by it. The first part is true but not the second.

I've got it. He'll describe me as a talking head in a body that can't move, like that guy in the *Star Trek* episode. You know, the one where, after a radiation explosion, all that remains of him is his head mounted on a brain wave–operated computer, on wheels no less. I've seen that episode many times. Seen all the *Star Treks* many times, like every other series in syndication. That episode is called "The Menagerie." Appropriate, don't you think, considering the nurses call this place "a zoo" when things get crazy busy, which is nearly all the time. You know the *Star Trek* description of me would be pretty good if a biomedical engineer would only hook up my jaw, and thus my brain, to my computer.

But maybe his kids don't watch TV or movies. Play computer games instead. Well, I plan to stop watching TV. Once I'm connected to my computer, I will never watch TV again. And I don't plan to play video games on my computer either. You see, I actually am more like Pollyanna than the talking head on *Star Trek* because I still have hope. Hope that my joystick will soon be connected to my computer and I will talk with people all over the world. Hope that soon I will write poetry. Hope that I won't lose the power in my jaw muscles, before I get connected. My jaw muscles have lasted for twenty-seven years since the rest of my body lost its power, and they'll definitely survive for the next year or so until I get connected.

So bring on the kids. Let them see the most ferocious animal in this fucking zoo.

Chapter 24

May 6, 2000

A long while passes.
All are staring downward
All are comfortably reflecting on Ruth
All except me.
I have never been so ill at ease.

Another Friend finally speaks.
She tells of helping "our Friend" smoke.
All eyes smile
Except mine.
All heads nod
Except mine.

The Friend finishes too soon for me
Then looks directly at me
Staring at me
Staring at me.

Chapter 25

October 1, 1998

Since his kids' visit, he's come to see me three nights in a row. Three nights in a row is a world's record. Probably a record that will last forever. And he's been hanging around for more than the standard medical three minutes.

I guess the three nights in a row is his way of thanking me for "permission" to bring his kids in to meet me. Probably thanking me even more for behaving myself when they were visiting. You would have been proud of me. I was a real lady, at least within reason. More Bacall or early Hepburn than de Havilland. And they found me waiting for them a full fifty feet from the hospital's main doors so I wouldn't be tempted. I didn't see them coming because I was facing the other way, drooling at the smokers surrounding the nine-foot perimeter of the hospital's main doors, where I had joined in a few minutes before, knowing doctors are always late.

They walked up quietly behind me, from the doctors' lot around the corner, I guess. The doc-who-wants-to-be-my-friend yelled, "Hi there" to give me time to pirouette my chair and face them in their final approach.

"Kids, this is my friend, Ruth," he glowed, paused, and gently encouraged, "Go ahead, introduce yourselves." They seemed confused and kept looking at my right hand, hoping, I guess, that I would extend it. The Doc jumped in with, "Remember Ruth can't lift her hand." They introduced themselves shyly, none of the confidence of the von Trapp children when stepping forward to introduce themselves. His kids just sort of nodded their heads when he introduced them, not knowing what to do with their right hands.

I have to admit that the visit with his kids was a nice distraction. Better than boredom. They were really quiet at first, looking at their feet a lot, like their Dad does, before lowering his eyes because he's embarrassed that he is going to tell me that he has to leave right away. At the beginning, they wouldn't speak unless I spoke directly to them, and then would only respond in a very polite whisper. But once I got them going with talking about movies, it was hard to stop them. They kept looking me straight in the eye, longer than their Dad ever has done, and soon became quite animated, like their Dad becomes in front of his students.

His kids have seen a lot of movies. And not just Disney, Spielberg, and Lucas. One told me his favourite movie was *The Great Escape,* and another told me the *Bridge on the River Kwai.* The third said, "My father likes *Gandhi* best and has made us watch it three times." I asked him what his favourite movie was. He said, "*Casablanca.*" I asked him what he thought *Casablanca* was about. He hesitated, stared down at his feet looking very serious and said, "Loyalty, devotion to great causes, and friendship." I've seen *Casablanca* dozens of times and always thought it was a love story.

They don't watch much TV, not even *Star Trek*. Don't seem to be into Atari games much either, except for something called "Where in the World is Carmen Sandiego?" which the oldest said is the only one they can play as long as they want. They're allowed to play two others, "Frogger" and "Donkey Kong," but as the oldest was quick to point out, they're only allowed thirty minutes a day on these and only because their Dad thinks it sharpens their hand-eye coordination.

My strange doctor-friend stood behind his kids when I was talking with them, grinning like the Cheshire Cat in a black jacket again. His children are obviously the centre of his life. He loves them very much. What a gift to be able to give love like that.

After about twenty minutes, the doc-who-wants-to-be-my-friend starts looking at his feet, indicating that he's embarrassed that he has to tell me that they have to leave. He tells his kids, "We better get going, there's homework to do. Say goodbye to Ruth."

They say "Good bye" much more confidently than they said "Hi." I told them they are welcome to visit with me anytime. The next time I'd show them the power in my power chair. The youngest beamed and said, "Cool." I refrained from promising I would knock down a doctor for them, even though I wanted to, because I assume I would have to be good again.

After they started walking away, I turned my chair and zoomed toward the front doors, hit the brakes, pirouetted. I caught the back of them about to round the corner of the hospital to "doctors' parking." For some reason, they stopped, turned around, and all waved.

I waited there about five minutes, which was quite hard, before trying to get someone to help me smoke a cig.

Tonight, his eyes have been on his feet ever since he got here. I know he needs to be somewhere else, but he doesn't want to appear unappreciative of my favour of meeting with his kids, at least he thinks I did him a favour, and it can do me no harm to ride that pony for a while. But finally I say, "Okay, I can see you're double-booked."

He finally apologizes for having "to leave so soon." Back to old times.

His standard existing ritual always concludes when he's at the door, poised to jump out with, "Is there anything you need, Ruth?" I always just stare at him. He always just leaves. But tonight, I whisper, and it has to be as loudly as I can because he's over at the door, "Hey, you born the identical day as me, I need my joystick hooked up to my computer."

He gives me that apologetic professional smile of his and says, "I'm sorry, Ruth, but my experience with computers is confined to helping my kids find 'Carmen Sandiego.'" He turns and heads for the door.

I quickly fill my lungs and whisper as loudly as I can, "Better go home to your kids."

He's out the door like a shot.

That's what I get for asking something and allowing myself to get hopeful. Just makes me feel like a piece of shit.

Suddenly he comes back. He stares at me with a determined look in his eyes that I've never seen before. He pulls a chair from across the room right beside my bed, and slowly draws the curtains around my bed.

"I'm sorry, Ruth. Please tell me about ..."

My computer, Doc.

Chapter 26

October 2, 1998

I call our Regional Biomedical Engineering Department and leave a message on the answering machine, requesting one of the engineers return my call. I prefix my name with "Doctor" to increase the likelihood of a response, perhaps even a prompt response. I hate playing the "Doctor" card, but I have played it before for family and friends. It is easier playing the "Doctor" card when speaking to an answering machine than when looking into someone's eyes.

Ruth's having to wait three years to have her joystick connected to her computer is obscene. What have we become? What kind of society makes people in Ruth's position wait three years to assist them, especially when a clear and simple strategy to help them readily exists, although I guess not readily accessible to everyone. Wait three years for assistance to read and write and learn and interact with the world. We do not delay medical treatment for three years, whether curative or to alleviate suffering. Why would we delay alleviating the suffering Ruth must daily endure by unnecessarily being excluded from a world of interacting with others? This is too cruel. Would not Ruth's overall health be promoted by her being able to use her amazing mind to communicate with others?

We did not learn about accommodating persons with disabilities in medical school. Actually, I don't remember learning anything at all about persons with disabilities, except how to determine "what is the lesion" and "where is the lesion." We were trained to be detectives, objectively gathering clues and evidence to establish the criminal lesion, rather than learning about, or caring about a person's experience of what the "lesion" means to them. I'm not sure there is much disability learning in medical school curricula now.

Ruth said there are only two biomedical engineers in our district hired to do the biophysical computations she needs to be able to use the joystick on her power chair to work her computer. Obviously, we need to hire more biomedical engineers, but that's not likely to happen in the current political climate. So I have to try to open the gate to one of the biomedical engineers for Ruth. Not that I believe in "queue jumping," for Ruth or anyone else. I would not even ask that one of my children be moved to a higher rung on a waiting list. However, I would, without hesitation call a colleague, who would without hesitation provide the "professional courtesy" of seeing my child in the clinic after regular office hours or meet my child in Emerg. Of course, this is queue jumping in a way, as somebody with no connection to these doctors would have to wait to be seen during regular clinic hours or in Emerg.

Physicians placate our consciences regarding professional courtesy with arguments like we are not making these other patients wait longer on the lists, as we are seeing the colleague's family members after hours, and isn't it true that people who know how to repair houses, or cars, will fix their friends' roofs, or sinks, or decks, or engines on weekends, while the rest of us wait our turn? I can't do anything but medicine. Nor can most doctors. So the only way we can help our family and friends is by staying late for each other's family and friends. I actually try hard to assuage my guilt this way, when I call the appropriate specialist to meet us in Emerg, rather than have family or friends endure the three or more hour wait to see the ER doctor, before the specialist that I knew was required and would be called is finally called.

I may be conflicted about having my kids cared for promptly in this way, but I am not *that* conflicted. I believe my obligation to my kids overrides my view on queue jumping.

It is more complicated with Ruth but not that much more complicated. Ruth is becoming my friend. Although Ruth is not a family member, I have no hesitation about calling a biomedical engineer, for her or anyone else in her situation. The injustice is that great. I am outraged by my health system. It's outrageous that Ruth does not have access to her computer.

So I feel no guilt calling the biomedical engineer. Well almost no guilt. I just hope he calls me back.

Chapter 27

May 6, 2000

They transfix my eyes with theirs.
Are they encouraging me
Or accusing me
Or just waiting for me
Patiently waiting for me.

I cannot bear their unswerving stare
Their patiently waiting for me
So I stand
And reach inside my jacket for a pocket that holds
A folded yellow sheet of lined paper
On which I had last night pencilled
Regret-riveted words.

All night I erased and wrote these words
Words that will inhibit my sleep
For the rest of my life
Words I worried I would have to speak today
Words I still worry I will not be able to speak
Today or ever
Words I have no choice but to speak
Today and always
Words that now disorient my eyes' focus
Words I know by heart.

I inhale a deep breath.
"It is not Ruth's life that I can share
For I knew little of Ruth's life
Neither can I share Ruth's death
For it is too painful for me to recount
But I can share Ruth's beauty
Beauty that beamed in every sound bite
I permitted her."

Chapter 28

November 25, 1999

One of the hospital chaplains was just here. No, I'm not in the midst of dying. No I'm not confessing many sins for salvation or to make a holy person blush. And, in case you haven't noticed, I haven't had much opportunity to sin lately. Unless you're such a prude you consider my occasional use of expressive language a sin.

Maybe the chaplains come to visit me to give me solace for not having the opportunity to sin. I mean if I don't get the opportunity to sin, I don't have the opportunity to demonstrate I have the strength to avoid sinning, let alone the opportunity to confess my sins, which the Catholic chaplains tell me is cathartic, before I tell them cathartic is a shit-laden word. And it's not like I'm busting to expunge thought-sins, which because I know I will never be able to commit them, I'm not sure count as sins at all. And I'm not referring to sexual thought-sins, rather thought-sins like incinerating all the asshole politicians who promote the tax breaks that break our health system.

It's in the job description of hospital chaplains to visit all hospital "admissions" soon after their "admissions," to see if we have anything to admit, and be able to absolve us of our admission just in case we die suddenly. Even if we're not reported to be at death's door, when of course they think it more likely to be successful in getting an admission out of us, they try to see us as soon as they learn we've been admitted.

They're hooked into the hospital's computer, I bet. If we've been admitted in the past, we may or may not have a record of successful admissions, which, in the case of chaplains, is a spiritually successful admission. I'm not sure if they keep these records on our hospital charts, or the chaplains have their own record-keeping system, which the chaplains may assume is more sacredly secure. Also from the chart, either the hospital's or the chaplain's, the chaplain may surmise whether or not it is likely that we have had the opportunity to sin since our last admission: in terms of days away, nature of our medical problem, nature of our spiritual problem, and personality in general. These factors may also be considered an indication of the likelihood and magnitude of sins that we could confess to and thus we could be absolved of. Of course, our propensity to confess on past admissions would also be an indicator as to whether or not we would confess and be absolved on this admission.

I know I'm sounding irreverent but it's hard not to in my situation. Nah, can't blame the situation, as I was irreverent long before I was immobile. The chaplains are all quick to tell me that they visit for my comfort, not for my confession. So I always tell them that they should get comfortable as well and to take the most comfortable chair in the room, which could be a commode or a recliner. Of course the recliners are too heavy to move and the commodes too personal, so after checking out the chairs-in-the-room status, the chaplains usually smile before returning to stand by my bed.

If I'm incarcerated for a while, sometimes two or three hospital chaplains will get the opportunity to visit me during my sentence. And as I have "no religious denomination" registered on my chart, as I spirited away my patriarchal religion confines in the sixties, chaplains of several Christian denominations are always eager to have the opportunity to try to re-religionize me to their alignment. I've also seen a rabbi a couple of times. I always allow the chaplains to talk on and on in the hushed, supportive, and at times syrupy sanctimonious tones they were taught in chaplain school. Better than boredom.

To be honest, I have to admit I enjoy chaplain visits. You see, over the years, I've developed a list of smartass questions that I throw at them, usually just before they're ready to leave. I bet myself whether or not this particular hospital chaplain will do a double take at my question, wondering whether he or she — there are several female chaplains now — has heard me right. They always hear it right, although sometimes they pretend they don't so they won't have to answer a faith-questioning question. I love watching the ones who do double takes, their eyes narrowing, honestly wondering if they heard me correctly, or whether I meant what I said, or understood the effect of what I said must have on a "man-of-the-cloth."

Recently I've developed a new send-off statement to immediately follow their "Have faith, Ruth." I tell them, "If your (I insert name of their religion here) will connect me to my computer, you can sign me right up for (again insert name of their religion here)." That provokes a pause or two before they get back in their sanctimonious pastoral posture until they give their sympathetic head nod and lip purse. Sympathy is not what I need, but they're just doing their job so I can't complain. It did piss me off when a chaplain once responded, "Faith can give you the strength to endure the wait." Give me a break. A very long one from you, I felt like saying, but of course didn't because I would never want to hurt the feelings of a "man-of-the-cloth."

You know, it's tempting to find faith when your soul aches. Tempting to find faith when the life you loved was whisked away and not-so-gradually replaced by a purgatory where you wait forever before you can ascend to Internetland. Especially if you have so much time on your hands to feel your soul ache, and not so much time on your hands before you get grimly reaped. So I must confess that I've swallowed my pride and seriously checked out faith after faith of whatever faith was the flavour of the hospital chaplain doing the comfort rounds on the neurology floor.

The chaplains of course were encouraged by the smell of a potential fresh convert and perhaps also by hope that my endangered soul could be saved even if there was no hope that my condemned body could be saved. The chaplains came to see me more and more frequently and talked to me longer and longer. Better than boredom. They seemed to no longer be afraid of me or, more important, of what I might say. My religion lessons, sometimes two or three times a day, really became an important part of my day. And, of course, I could avoid all distractions and put all my energy and time to think about religion between lessons.

I really did take exploring faith seriously, I have to confess. I also have to confess that this Jesus guy is a really cool dude. What a rebel. Great one-liners. He said something like instead of babbling your faith in many words in front of many people, keep your faith within and speak to God like you were in a closet where no one can hear you. Talk about perfect for me. Confucius was cool, too. Also rolled off lots of one-liners. And some really smartass ones at that. He also had a social conscience and talked about doing unto others as you would have them do unto you, like Jesus did. Well I can't do anything for others. But I would if I could. Lao Tzu gave me lots to think about. However the rabbis and Buddhists were rare, compared with the priests and ministers, so most of the time I was in Christian mode. Then I heard from a nurse on the ward about her "Circle of Friends." I think I decided to become a Quaker right then and there.

It's not that I never knew about Quakers before. I've seen *Friendly Persuasion* with Gary Cooper and Dorothy McGuire many times. Pacifism and love and all that good stuff. Beautiful title track, too, if you like romantic songs, which I do. And of course Grace Kelly was a Quaker in *High Noon*, again with Gary Cooper but Cooper wasn't a Quaker this time. In fact, he shot a lot of people, but they were bad guys and he was the sheriff. Grace Kelly even shot a bad guy, too, in order to save her husband (Gary Cooper), so I guess you could consider her violence a love crime. I of course knew about the role Quakers played in the "underground railway," having grown up not far from the northern terminus in Dresden, Ontario, where there are all kinds of commemorative plaques and stuff. But what I learned from the nurse, that convinced me that being a Quaker was right for me, was that there are no sermons in a Quaker service, or meeting as they call it. Lots of silence, rather than sermonizing. I'm into that.

Chapter 29

October 2, 1998

My assistant comes into the Clinic and tells me, "The engineer you're waiting to hear from is on the line."

I dash to my office after apologizing to the woman waiting for me in the examining room, but remembering that I forgot to apologize to the women waiting for me in the waiting room. I'll do that later. I need to focus on the biomedical engineer. I have rehearsed what I need to say him many times, and again rapidly rehearse my plea of Ruth's case one more time on the way to my office. I pick up the phone, take a deep breath, and release the hold button.

"Hello, Sir. Thank you for returning my call so quickly."

I hear a friendly deep voice say, "No problem, Doctor" and then tell me his name.

I rapidly tell Ruth's story without taking a breath so the biomedical engineer has no space to interrupt me with "I can't help you." I am quick to insist that I am not asking him to see Ruth in place of someone else. Rather "I am hoping you can see Ruth after hours, and I would be happy to pay you for your time and inconvenience." I quickly add "and expertise of course," and even quicker "at an overtime rate of course," and "I would consider it a personal favour and —"

He jumps in before I can embarrass myself further with "Don't you think that every parent with financial means whose child has cerebral palsy or a neuromuscular condition offers to pay me to see their child after hours?"

"I'm sorry, I didn't realize —"

"They all want their child in computerized education, rather than falling farther and farther behind kids their age."

"I'm sorry —"

"Many parents without the financial means promise to beg, borrow, or steal to pay me."

"I'm sorry —"

"I stopped returning phone calls two years ago. The only reason I'm returning your call is because you're a physician."

I need to regroup my thoughts. I pause, then say, "I'm sorry to have bothered you. I should have better appreciated your situation." But this is my one chance for Ruth so I have to keep trying. I change my strategy. "Isn't there anything *we* can do for Ruth?"

He pauses and quietly responds in a sympathetic voice, "I'm sorry, she'll have to be patient."

Chapter 30

December 10, 1999

I've got another butt bedsore. The nurse who visits the group home when the need arises has me lying on my stomach all day, bare-assed to the world. It's not that I'm em-bare-assed. How could I be after all these years? It's just a royal pain-in-the-ass because I have to stare down at my bedsheets through a rubber doughnut thing that holds my forehead and chin off the sheets so I don't suffocate, when I would much rather than be in my power chair staring at the sometimes more stimulating TV down the hall. This ass-to-the-air thing is worth it though, if the "fresh air" stops the damn foul bedsore from getting infected again.

The nurse feels bad about me getting bedsores. She knows I wouldn't get bedsores, at least not as often or as bad, if the staff in the group home had the time to turn my body more frequently. I know she knows because I heard her tell an attendant more than once that they need to turn me more frequently to stop the skin on my scrawny ass from being crushed by my butt bones. The nurse didn't exactly say "scrawny ass" but that's what she meant, and my ass is scrawny because my ass muscles have degenerated because the connections to my spinal cord no longer work. And it's not the attendant's fault. I know that because I heard an attendant once say to the nurse she would like to turn me more often but there really was no extra time to do this sort of thing because of the staff cuts.

The nurse once told me that she'd look into getting me a computerized air mattress with an air compressor that inflates and deflates various areas of the mattress to decompress my body's pressure off the skin over my bony butt at regular intervals. One of the patients here has one of these automatic air mattresses, but he had to buy it himself. I know because I rolled right up to him and asked him straight out how he rated. I wonder how the nurse knows I can't afford to buy a power mattress myself. I hope the nurse comes through with a computerized air mattress cause I'm afraid of bedsores. In the meantime, the nurse said, it was up to the attendants to find the time to turn me.

It's not that I'm in any physical pain from the bedsore. I mean I can't feel the damn thing. It's just that I'm really afraid the bedsore will get infected again. And the infection will spread through my entire body again. And I will wind up in Emerg again. And Emerg is a very dangerous place for someone "like me."

You see, a year and a half ago, I became very septic from an infected bedsore. By the time they got me to Emerg, I was so weak that I couldn't open my eyes or even my mouth. The Emerg doctors thought I was unconscious. This should not be surprising because, not only could I not open my eyes, nor speak, nor nod my chin to indicate that I heard them speaking to me, but I couldn't feel them pinching the hell out of my arm, so I couldn't "respond to painful stimuli." It appears that this "respond to painful stimuli" is a very important sign of consciousness. At least it's an important sign of consciousness for people who can feel their arms when they're conscious. But for people "like me" who can't feel pinching or pin pricking, it is a more than useless test of consciousness. It is a dangerous test of consciousness.

Although I couldn't feel the ER docs pinching me, I could sure hear them talking about me. I could hear them debating "death with dignity now" or possible existence in a "persistent vegetative state" — perhaps for a long time — connected to a ventilator — in their "Expensive Care unit." One of them worried that my being on a ventilator in Expensive Care for a long time would deny the bed to someone who could recover with a higher "quality of life." I hate this "quality-of-life" bullshit. "Quality-of-life scores" can trap people "like me" in lethal traps. Who are they to determine my "quality of life"?

I really thought they were going to let me "die with dignity" right then and there, curtained off from help, where no one could hear my heart screaming I want to live. I want to live no matter what.

Because, as I'm sure you would now agree, the ER can be such a dangerous place for someone "like me." I have thought about asking a friend to write me an "Advance Directive" like I saw on *Chicago Hope*, which would easily be the best doctor show on TV if George Clooney was in it. Anyway, on this episode of *Hope*, a fifty-something man was in a terrible car accident and is brought by ambulance to Emerg with no signs of life. His face is terribly bruised and swollen. His eyeballs bulge out like a bullfrog's. I think they said he probably had brain damage. Anyway, the ER docs continue the CPR the ambulance guys had started, and put a tube down his throat so they can ventilate him better with an "Ambu bag" until they could get him on a ventilator. While all this is going on, a nurse goes through his wallet and finds a card with an "Advance Directive" indicating that "no heroic measures" are to be done for him if he cannot say this for himself. The ER docs stopped ventilating him.

My "Advance Directive" would say exactly the opposite: I want everything be done for me to keep me alive, no matter what, including "heroic measures." But, just as I was going to go the "Advance Directive" route, I heard that "Advance Directives" apparently can be "open to interpretation" by the doctors because they could argue that it was not possible for the patient to have precisely predicted their condition when the

"Advance Directive" was signed, such as the exact situation in which the doctors find the patient when "heroic measures" like long-term ventilation are being considered. So, as the doctors don't know if I would have signed the "Advance Directive" in the way I did if I had known I would be in the circumstances in which the docs now find me in Emerg, they can determine whether or not I get "heroic measures." I began worrying that my written words could be used against me to allow my "death with dignity." You would worry about this, too, if you had a previous Emerg experience like mine. Fortunately I learned about a better alternative than an "Advance Directive." Sometimes good things come to those who wait in hospital clinic waiting rooms all afternoon.

Last time I was in a waiting room, I overheard two of the other waiters talking about this new thing called "Life Story Decision Making." You write the names of friends who know your life story on a special card you keep in your wallet. These friends would have to know you well enough to know what decisions you would make for yourself if you were able to do so. Most important, you need to have a great deal of trust in these friends that they will try to make the decisions for you that you would want them to make, but stand up to doctors who might believe the decision they are making for you is inappropriate. Three women whom I obviously trust have already written their names and phone numbers on the special card that I now have in my wallet in the sack on the back of my chair.

I'm also going to ask my doctor-friend if he would add his name to my trusted-ones card. I know you're thinking he doesn't know me very well. You're right. I don't think we've talked more than a dozen times, and they were usually very short times, of course. But he was outraged when I told him about the "death with dignity" debate in Emerg. And he definitely knows I want to live no matter what. And the main reason I need my doctor-friend's name and numbers on my card is because his MD degree is my best defence against "death with dignity." Doctors will have to listen to him when he tells them I want to live no matter what. He's a member of their club. They won't be able to browbeat him like they will try to do to the women on my list. Rather they'll respect his decision for me because he's one of them.

To be completely honest with you, I've already had the woman who wrote her name last on my list write his name and phone numbers under hers. You know, his home number is actually listed in the phone book. She thought that "very strange" for a doctor. I told her, "You don't know the half of the strangeness of this doctor."

I will ask his permission to be on my list next time I see him.

Chapter 31

October 2, 1998

I wonder what it would cost to take Ruth to the States. Many Canadians now go to the States to buy prompt healthcare. Canadians with the financial means, that is. They don't hesitate to cross the border for a next-day MRI there, as part of their medical work here. Wealthy Canadians diagnosed there are treated sooner here. Some wealthy Canadians go to the States for quicker access to surgery after their initial medical work here. If you can buy prompt investigation and treatment in the States, I assume you can also buy prompt biomedical engineer services. The border is only an hour away. And I know that medical clinics catering to Canadians exist near the border — some, believe it or not, in retail strip malls as soon as you cross the border.

Being connected to her computer is all Ruth asks for in life. Not much to ask for. A few hours of a biomedical engineer's time would permit Ruth to unwind the thousands of hours of thought and creativity stored in her mind since her freedom-to-engage watch stopped almost twenty years ago. A few hours of a biomedical engineer's time would release Ruth from her solitary confinement to thousands of hours of the freedom to engage many minds and hearts. A few hours of a biomedical engineer's time would allow Ruth's wonderful mind and heart to finally be heard, instead of Ruth being forced to listen to the limitations of TV all day.

I know for certain that if any of my children had to wait like Ruth, I would immediately take them to the States, no matter what. I would find the money. I would find the time. But Ruth is not my child. Finding the money would be easier than finding the time. No, that's a cop-out. I can't use my usual too-busy-with-patients or too-busy-with-kids cards to trump Ruth, the way I use my obligations to my patients and children to absolve me of everything else. I could hire one of the caregivers at Ruth's home to take her to the States. I am sure they would like to make some extra money on a day off. They must be paid only minimum wage. I can set up everything with the American biomedical engineer on the phone. I really should look into sending Ruth to the States.

Chapter 32

February 5, 2000

That bedsore I was telling you about resolved after a few weeks on oral antibiotics and air. No need for ERs and Drs. And I have something even more important and even more personal to tell you about — if you believe something is more personal than my vulva. Okay, here we go.

I am in love.

I am completely and so deeply in love that I am about to burst. I have found the soul mate I sought for so many years. TV clichés, I know. But I have hoped to feel these clichés for so long that I don't care if you think I'm getting soft and ruining my reputation. These clichés are exactly how I feel. I have thought about finding love constantly. And I have had lots of lonely time on my hands to think about love. So many silent hours spent thinking about even the possibility of love for me. And now I am in love.

He listens to me so eagerly, longing to learn me. He speaks to me so earnestly, always looking into my eyes. I love the way he smoothes my hair from my forehead with fingers as gentle as feathers. I love the way he moves my drinking straw back to my lips when it goes amiss. Adjusting it just so. Asking me to make sure it's just where I want it. I love the way he lovingly tickles my chin. I love the love in his eyes when he touches me anywhere. Each caress of his fingers smoothes away years of loneliness. I have never been so alive.

He calls me his calcedony because, he says, I'm beautiful to the core though just a little crusty on the surface. Not bad, eh? Okay, I showed him my bookends. He calls them my computer ends. He's very funny.

His name is Alex, but I call him Fred. Fred had a stroke. The left side of his body doesn't move. He uses a chair, but not a power chair like mine. Even if he had a power chair, he wouldn't be able to keep up with me. But then few can.

Fred writes me poetry. He writes me poem after poem, and although his speech is a little slurry, he lovingly reads them to me when we're alone in my room. As soon as I'm connected to my computer, I will write Fred poem after poem. Poem after poem of the love I've collected in my heart for so many years. Poem after poem of the love pumping my heart every second I am awake. And I am exquisitely awake.

Wait just a sec, there's an attendant coming into my room. I'll tell you more about Fred later.

Chapter 33

February 17, 2000

A still new attendant comes into my room smiling as usual, and heads straight for my pillows, saying, "Good evening, Ruth" on the way. She puffs the pillows without moving my head, as she's been trained to do, and starts performing her other evening maintenance manoeuvres on me.

She starts by taking off my makeup with makeup remover, then clarifying my skin with special emollients to make sure no sign of age creeps into my face. Just kidding, of course. I don't wear makeup. I hardly ever wore makeup, even in my preconfinement days. Why would I now, and who has time to put it on or take it off, so I'm just fine thank-you-very-much. But she does brush my teeth very gently with a sponge toothbrush. And she does change my piss bag, very discreetly I might add. She does make sure I haven't pooped myself. That's easy to do. And finally she turns me a bit. On days when I'm lucky — that is, when she has the time — she gives me a full-body sponge bath. I love the smell of the soap and the feel of the warm water on my face.

Tonight she says, "Ruth, are you going for a train ride?"
"What?"
"A train ride. I heard that an engineer's coming to see you next week."
"What? When?"
"Tuesday, I think."
I freeze. I try to speak but can't. I try again but can't. She's heading for the door.

I shriek, "Stop."

I scared her but she stopped.

"What about the engineer?"

"I think they said something about an engineer coming to assess you." She smiles and leaves. The word "assess" sends a glass splinter through me. For the first time in my life, I am truly afraid. I've waited so long for this engineer to come, but now I'm terrified to see him. News too good to be true usually is. There'll probably be a glitch. I've had lots of time to think about glitches like what if my jaw muscles aren't working well enough anymore? Or what if I get another bedsore and I'm in the hospital when he comes. How long will it be before he can come back? Do I drop to the bottom of his list? You can see why I am truly terrified.

Chapter 34

May 6, 2000

Ruth gave me so much
Asked so little
Received much less.
All Ruth wanted was to have the joystick on her wheelchair —
Sorry, "power chair" —
Connected to her computer.
Ruth was denied even that
Denied even that
By our supposedly wonderful health and social support systems
Denied even that by me.

It was too much trouble for me
To take the time to make sure Ruth had what she needed
Even too much trouble to take the time
To visit Ruth at the group home
Or even call her at the group home
And ask an attendant to place the phone beside Ruth's ear.
Ruth was just too low on my radar screen to be seen
Unless she almost ran me over with her power chair.

Chapter 35

February 22, 2000

The biomedical engineer gently places my chin into this cold metal cup he calls a transducer. The cup is connected by thin black and red wires to a little black box that looks just like the Geiger counters they use in old movies to test for radiation: a little glass windshield over trembling red needle and all. I don't hear any Geiger counter static though. And I sure don't want to give this guy any static. Heaven is in his hands. I'm on my very best behaviour.

I ask, "Hey, Mr. Biomedical Engineer, do you think I'm hot?" Whoops.

I'm not sure he got my double meaning as he remains in his very serious decorum, which is probably a good thing, but after a few seconds, he smiles and reminds me to move my jaw only when he asks me to. I still don't think he got my joke and have to keep telling myself, be good, Ruth, and "you can do it, Ruth" in my best Cheech Marin, both, of course, silently because I'm no ventriloquist, and I am certainly not going to move my jaw again and piss this guy off.

He's been here for over an hour. It's hard for me to be good this long. Especially when I'm really scared, and pretending so hard not to look scared at all, and pretending so hard to be a "proper lady," as I keep telling myself in Audrey Hepburn's Eliza Doolittle voice.

Finally, he starts gathering his stuff to leave, putting his wires and electric meters and other stuff back in his case. Then he stands, walks to the door, and smiles, and says, "Goodbye, Ruth."

I can't just let him leave without knowing when he'll come back, so I try to stop him with,

"Yo, Mr. Biomedical Engineer, when do we hook up?" in my "Rocky" voice.

It stopped him.

He smiles again, but apologetically this time.

"I'm sorry, Ruth, you'll have to be patient."

Chapter 36

April 27, 2000

I have another butt bedsore. The nurse has me lying on my stomach all day, ass-naked to the world, "to let the air get at it." They have been applying the usual poultices, powders, and other potions to try to get rid of the damn thing. Even started me on antibiotics, which, of course, means they think it is infected. The worst part about this bedsore is I can't let Fred into my room. Not because I'm modest, of course. Too late for that. It's just that I'm sure the bedsore looks awful. And I think it's starting to smell.

I overheard the nurse whispering to an attendant that if the bedsore looks worse tomorrow, she's going to send me to Emerg. The nurse didn't mention this to me. Maybe because she knows I have a morbid fear of Emerg, and she doesn't want me to worry. But even nurses forget that quads can hear as well as anyone else and better than most in here, so I'm really worried.

I hope the nurse calls my neurologist, so he can admit me directly to the ward, so I don't have to spend the whole day in Emerg waiting to be seen by an ER doc before I can be referred to a neurologist and admitted. I'm going to ask the nurse about avoiding Emerg when she comes in tomorrow, but I really wouldn't mind being admitted to hospital if the damn thing's infected. Just as long as I don't have to be seen in Emerg first. If the damn bedsore's bacteria spreads through my body again, and the total body infection makes me look unconscious to the Emerg docs again, it will be the "death with dignity" debate again, and this time I may not survive it.

Relax. Deep breaths. This time, I have a card in my wallet with the names and phone numbers of those I trust to tell the docs that I want to live no matter what. I also have a note on my chart directing them to find the card in my wallet if any "substitute decision making" is required. But what if the nurses are too busy to look for my wallet in my bag on the back of my chair? What if, by the time the group home nurse decides to send me to Emerg, I'm too weak to be put in my chair with my bag on back, or even to make sure that my bag comes to Emerg with me and that someone knows to look for my wallet inside? What if the ER staff finds my wallet and the card but can't reach any of my trusted ones? What if they don't even try to reach them?

I wonder if I should ask tonight's attendant to call the numbers on my list, just in case. It wouldn't hurt. I need to alert my trusted ones that I may be going to Emerg, that I may be in danger. It wouldn't hurt to let them know that they may soon be on-call for me, to make sure I don't get discarded in Emerg. To insist I am more than a bloody gauze, plastic suture tray, or other waste left over from helping those with a better "quality of life."

I'm so worried I'm having trouble breathing. I must relax. Breathe deeply.

I've probably had bedsores like this one before that have healed without getting me septic. I don't want to overreact. I don't want to waste the time of the people on my card or waste the caregiver's time required for her to track them down. I don't want to be accused of crying wolf.

I will ask the caregiver next time she comes in to put my sack beside my face in my bed. Just in case. She'll think I'm crazy, but as she probably already thinks so, I have nothing to risk. I won't bother anyone else unless it is absolutely necessary. I have my reputation to consider.

Chapter 37

1330 h, April 30, 2000

Yet another conference. I hate being away from my kids, even for two days. Airplanes are very claustrophobic. I fly home this evening, but before that, in about an hour, I will give the talk I was asked to give, the core message of which half the audience has heard me urge before. A message consistent with the views of many of this audience; but many others, including those supposed to be responsible for health and social policy, cannot, or will not, hear my arguments because they cannot, or will not, see beyond the blinkers of budget-balancing imperatives in the age of "fixed" health and social resources.

I patiently wait at the back of the convention hall for my turn to address the audience. I always sit at the back, so I can get up, stretch, and walk around, frequently to the bathroom, without disturbing anyone. There are about five hundred people sitting in front of me today on a flat conventional hall floor, rather than an amphitheatre.

The speaker presenting before me is called to the podium. I see heads of the audience members turn left, and the occasional person stands to see her as she rolls her electric wheelchair to beside the stage. I also stand. The audience members softly murmur to each other. There is a ramp to the stage, at the bottom of which she waits, while someone leans over, discussing something with her. The podium is moved slightly, and the woman rapidly ascends the stage and quickly turns her chair to face us. The moderator of this afternoon's program bends over her, clipping a microphone to the collar of her yellow blouse. The speaker softly says into the microphone,

"I am the healthiest person I know."

All murmuring stops. The audience is silent. "The healthiest person I know" surprises us because the speaker is quadriplegic. The speaker continues, explaining that she is the healthiest person she knows, even though she has a little bit less DNA on one of her chromosomes than most people have. She tells us that having a little less DNA on this chromosome results in her having no power in most of her muscles.

I walk partway up the left side of the amphitheatre to see her better. I see calmly engaging eyes, fiercely compelling us through large rimless glasses that seem to magnify her quiet intensity. I see that she is about my age. I see that her right hand is Velcroed to her chair's right armrest. I see that her right hand holds a small joystick. I see the back and seat of her chair periodically raising, lowering, and tilting, to rotate the pressure off her skin's weight-bearing points.

She speaks so powerfully in her gentle whisper, crediting her wonderful health to three "social determinants of health" — two "social determinants" from the World Health Organization: "education" and "financial means." The third she added herself, "love."

The speaker tells us of the importance of her partner's love in making each of her days healthy in many ways. The speaker tells us of the importance of her love for her partner in infusing energy and commitment through her arteries; the importance of her love for her partner in keeping her healthy to carry on her writing. The speaker says her partner is always with her, supportively, spiritually, lovingly, then looks at a modestly smiling woman in the front row, about her age.

She goes on to describe how her parents' love and adequate financial means permitted her an education where pages could be turned and doors opened, both physically and metaphorically. She acknowledges that her parents were able to purchase all the measures of accommodation she required that eventually allowed her to become an educator and advocate, and to use the tremendous amount of knowledge, sensitivity, and understanding gleaned from the hundreds of thousands of pages she read along the way. She explains how her parents' love and financial means opened the world to her in other ways. They were able to take her places by paying for the assistance and accommodation she required. Her parents were able to immerse her in a world that is denied most people with disabilities. Having been engaged by that world of books and people and places, she now engages us with the wisdom of her words and the example of her being, just as her voice has been heard all over the world.

The speaker tells us that when she takes a break from teaching and writing advocacy articles, she enjoys writing poetry. She writes by speaking into a microphone attached to her computer, and her words are transcribed into text through software called "Dragon." I immediately think of Ruth. I'm sure Ruth has mentioned that this "Dragon" software is already loaded on her computer.

The speaker goes on to describe how Apple has developed many disability-friendly software programs, so that all people with disabilities who have computers will have access to the Internet. The software can be designed to accommodate the needs of any particular person. She gave the example of the microphone near her mouth that was currently attached to the conference centre's amplification system. Ruth had told me all about this software.

The speaker says she will end her talk by reading the list of names and causes of death of persons killed by recent government cutbacks* to programs that assist people with disabilities. A woman starved to death because the funding was cut for someone to check in on her to make sure she was buying groceries and eating. A man was burned to death because he was placed into a bath of scalding water by a new attendant who was less costly to the system. Many names and atrocities follow. With each name, my heart hears a bell chime, and I imagine a candle being lit. By the time she finishes her talk, the stage seemed carpeted with candles of compassion, of equality, of purpose, of solidarity. Through her clip-on microphone, she has spoken the most powerful words I have ever heard.

The audience explodes in ovation. All are standing now. I think of Ruth. I must tell Ruth about this amazing woman. You know, I have not seen Ruth for a while. She must be doing well.

Chapter 38

May 6, 2000

Ruth's last sentence to me began with "I am in love."
In an excited voice I had not previously heard her use
Her voice
Her real voice.

Then realizing her formidable façade had cracked open enough
To allow me a look inside her sensitivity
She quickly rolled her eyes
And switched to her Mae West voice
"Why don't you come up and see me sometime
And I'll tell you all about him."

Then she smiled
As if in recognition of her almost letting me in
But not quite
Pirouetted her chair
And called out her room number as she sped off
Irrepressible as always.
I yelled I would come up after my clinic
But I never did get up to see her.

Ruth made our lives more beautiful
Because Ruth lived as long as she did
Though many years less than Ruth wanted to live
Many years less than Ruth could have lived.

Chapter 39

2210 h, April 30, 2000

Because of my flight connections, I won't arrive home until after midnight, as per usual after I speak at a conference. During the cross-country plane ride home, my mind has been rewinding the powerful speaker's passionate words over and over. I am riveted by "I am the healthiest person I know," "education, financial means … and love." But now I find myself back in primary school, to grade six, when our teacher had us all prepare "public speeches," which were really speeches for the teacher, and, in retrospect, for each other.

Sheila Heller was the shortest girl in our class. All the guys liked Sheila because she was a tomboy, funny, and of course cute. She also had the coolest last name, Heller. We could yell Heller in the schoolyard all we wanted and be free from the peril of getting the strap for swearing. We would flaunt the ability, and yell Heller right in front of strict teachers on yard duty. Sheila's public speech began with, "My name is Sheila Heller and I'm going to speak on Helen Keller." We broke up in hilarity, assuming that Heller had created a fictional character rhyming with her name. Sheila Heller on Helen Keller. But our rowdiness evaporated as Heller told us about a girl almost our age, who, as an infant, became deaf and blind from a virus. The doctors told her parents she was "mentally retarded" and should be institutionalized. Sheila told us how Helen Keller's parents loved her very much and wanted Helen to stay with them, so they hired a teacher to help Helen and live with them in their mansion. Sheila described how Helen's teacher, Annie Sullivan, who was almost blind herself, helped Helen learn to speak and read Braille. Sheila told us Helen Keller became a public speaker and writer.

I remember showing my children the film version of Helen Keller's relationship with Annie Sullivan, *The Miracle Worker*, on one of our "Thursday Night at the Movies." If Helen Keller's parents had not possessed the love and financial means to hire a one-on-one teacher, Helen Keller would have been confined for life in an institution, a life with no communication with anyone.

I keep thinking about the speaker. I keep thinking about Ruth. I have not seen Ruth for quite a while. I guess she has been well. At least not back in hospital, or she or someone else would have let me know. All Ruth wants is to be able to communicate through her computer. If Ruth only had the financial means, she would have been able to engage with the world for many years now.

I must go and see Ruth at her group home as soon as I can. You know, I've never been to Ruth's group home. Never once.

Chapter 40

0120 h, May 1, 2000

I quietly open the front door to my home. My feet magnetically move to my answering machine. No red light flashing, but there is a note beside it from my youngest: "Hospital has been looking for you Dad going to bed."

I'm not on call. Must be some mistake.

I phone the Hospital and page the resident on call. A sleepy voice answers, "Hello."

"I'm sorry to wake you up, but are you looking for me?"

"No. You're not covering tonight are you?"

"No. Again I'm sorry for waking you."

The Hospital must have called me by mistake. Some confusion now rectified.

I walk to my bedroom, throw my jacket on the chair, kick off my shoes, and fall back on the bed, eyes are already shut.

I wake to the phone ringing.

"Yes."

"Ruth's in trouble," a woman's voice whispers urgently. "Please come to the hospital right away."

I hear a dial tone. I see that it's 3:00 a.m.

I quickly put on my jacket and shoes, and speed to the Hospital. I park illegally at the ER doors and run in. The woman at ER reception tells me Ruth is not there, and hasn't been since she came on at seven. Good. Ruth must have been admitted. I ask the receptionist which room Ruth is in. Her computer is taking too long. I run up the stairs and down the hall to Intensive Care.

The nurse at the desk seems to be expecting me. She appears frightened. She doesn't say anything. Instead her eyes move from mine to look down at the index finger of her right hand. It is pointing to a draped-off area at the Unit's far end, about fifty metres away. I turn my head and see incandescent curtains projecting ominous shadows. I turn my body to dash there, but the nurse grips my right wrist hard, while gently whispering in a soothing but frightened voice, "Why don't you stay here with me until they're finished."

I extricate my wrist and run. I stop outside the curtain, clench the curtain's right edge and take a deep breath. These drapes will not be Ruth's shrouds. I fling open the curtains — to horror. Ruth. Oh, Ruth.

Her body is swollen to a huge black balloon, knotted at her neck, elbows, and wrists by a sadistic birthday party clown. Ruth's closed eyes bulge to black tennis balls. Her chin is gone. I see a black Michelin Man.

Without deviating my gaze, I quickly try to diagnose what has happened to Ruth. I work hard to force all emotion to the periphery so that I can objectively analyze Ruth's situation and come up with a treatment strategy. Her skin must be blackened by necrotizing bacteria that have quickly disseminated from a bedsore, and are now spreading their gas bubbles into Ruth's skin. The gas is strangulating the blood vessels not only in her skin but likely all her organs. We have to act fast or she will die. This is much worse than when bacteria last spread throughout Ruth's body from a bedsore and made her look unconscious in Emerg.

There are three IVs with antibiotics running. Ruth is bleeding from all the IV puncture sites, as well from around her mouth where the end of the tracheal tube was inserted, which means there are no platelets and other clotting factors left because the bacteria have caused disseminated intravascular coagulation and the blood-clotting components are being consumed by clots forming within her bloodstream and depositing in her kidneys, liver, and other organs. Ruth's urinary catheter bag is empty, so her kidneys are likely shut down, either from clots or from low blood pressure from all the fluid collecting in her skin and her abdomen. Ruth is on a ventilator. Good. Her heart is beating rapidly but regularly.

The left periphery of my underwater vision sees a woman sitting by Ruth's bed. Her shoulders are shuddering. Tears stream down her face. The right periphery of my underwater vision sees the ICU doc. He was one of my students, a Monday Night Medical Humanities regular. He is standing beside an elevated medication tray, drawing drugs into syringes.

He is not surprised to see me. Indeed seems to be expecting me. When I turn to him, he lifts his head and acknowledges me, sympathetically nodding his head as if to say, "Yes, it's too bad" and "Yes, I know you know her." He then goes back to preparing the syringes.

Hollowness expands within me, vacuuming me downward. I can stop this. Ruth wants "to live no matter what." I look hard at Ruth. I work hard to see Ruth. I work hard to breathe. I am drowning in what I see.

I turn to my former student. "You're not going to disconnect her are you?"

He puts his left hand on my right shoulder and stares at me with a sympathetic look. Finally he says, "I'm sorry" and goes back to his syringes.

I tell him firmly, "Ruth wants to live no matter what."

He does not lift his eyes or acknowledge what I have said.

I repeat, "Ruth wants to live no matter what."

Still no acknowledgement.

I calmly cradle my arms in a beseeching posture and say, "Ruth has made it very clear to me and others that she wants everything to be done for her no matter what." He finally lifts his head and stares at me but says nothing.

"Ruth wants to live no matter what," I repeat again.

He sighs, reaches out and grips my right upper arm and stares at me. He sighs again and gently whispers, "There's nothing of Ruth left."

"How can you be so sure?"

He firms his fingers on my right arm and turns me to face Ruth. He says, "Look."

Now I'm supposed to put my body between his body and Ruth's body. Ruth trusts me to do just that. Now I'm supposed to insist that Ruth remain on the ventilator. But the visage in Ruth's bed bears no resemblance to Ruth, bears little resemblance to human form. My hand goes to the hilt of my sword, but I keep its blade in its scabbard. I need to think. I need to calmly think. I take a deep breath. I take another deep breath. I am a doctor, trained to be calm, trained to be objective. I am a doctor, experienced in life-and-death situations. I am also Ruth's friend. I know that if Ruth could speak she would say that she wants to remain on life support. I know that Ruth wants me to demand that she remain on life support. Ruth wants me to refuse to move. Ruth wants me to make them call security. To make them take this to court.

I stare at Ruth. I know what I must do. But instead I place my lips where Ruth's left ear should be and plead, "Ruth, give me some sign. Twitch an eyelid. Twitch the skin on your chin. Please, Ruth, show him that there's something left. Please, Ruth. Please."

Chapter 41

May 6, 2000

Ruth was beautiful to her core
Is beautiful to her core
Like the bookends that stood beside her computer
The bookends that now stand beside my computer.

Ruth explained many things to me
Perhaps beginning with explaining that her bookends are calcedonies
Crusty-surfaced rocks
That open to amethyst
Agate
Onyx
Chrysoprase
To geodes of all shapes and sizes.
Ruth told me calcedonies can become jewellery
Amulets
Sculpture
Paperweights
For into each calcedony's core
Millennia have poured their alloyed amazement.
Ruth told me that calcedonies can endow wisdom
Courage
Healing powers
Spiritual powers
That each calcedony is unique

Wonderfully one of a kind
Like Ruth.
That each calcedony is beautiful
Wonderfully beautiful
Like Ruth.

I will try to share Ruth's beauty
By telling her story
As she requested me to do
Within my limitation
Of lived experience
Within my limitation of skill
Within my limitation of trust.
And I will introduce Ruth as my friend
To whomever I tell her story
My friend who wanted to be a poet
But is a poem
My friend to whom I failed to be
A friend.

Epilogue

Spring 2005

They think I have MS. My family doctor, the neurologist she referred me to, the subspecialist neurologist he referred me to, the neuroophthalmologist she referred me to all think I have MS. They speak to me in noncommittal medical euphemisms rather than "burdening" me with a diagnosis that is not yet "definitive," but they think I have MS. I welcome their avoidance of a not yet "definitive" diagnosis that will be so definitive for me.

I have developed an intermittent paralysis of the small muscles that control the movement of my right eyeball. Small muscles, like eye muscles, I understand, may weaken first with MS. Two or three times a day, in ten- to fifteen-minute intervals, the walls spin because my right eyeball is "rotating out of control" like an out-of-control hand-held camera, and I find myself plastered against the nearest wall. At least I am told that my right eyeball is "rotating out of control," never having been able to observe this phenomenon myself, as I cannot see anything during my right eyeball's delinquency. Eventually I learn to cover up my right eye so I can see through my still well-behaved left eye, albeit not stereoscopically, but my left eye cannot see my right eyeball rotate because my right eye is covered up by my right hand.

Covering up my right eye allows me to ignore what is going on. Covering up my right eye allows me to cover up from my clinical colleagues what is going on in someone on whom they rely and require to function at one hundred percent capacity now and in the future. Although none of my colleagues ever comments, those who observe me standing tipsy or intermittently wobbling along the Hospital's walls from our offices to the Clinic with my right hand covering my right eye know something is going on, but politely ignore that something is going on. I am grateful for their feigned lack of observation. Covering up my right eye also allows me to cover up what is going on from my patients. Although the occasional woman who witnesses me struggling to look in her eyes with my left eye while scrawling her presenting symptoms and history with my untrained left hand on her chart knows something is going on, I never see mistrust in their eyes. That would be too hard.

Of course I am sent for an MRI. For those of you who have not had the privilege, you deposit your clothes, wallet, and "any loose metal" (as opposed to metal in a replacement joint, cardiac pacemaker, or intrauterine contraceptive device) in a locker outside the magnet's room. Then, in a standard open-backed, greyish-blue hospital gown, you lie on a greyish-white slab that feels like cold steel, but must be plastic or fibreglass, considering the slab with you on it will be rolled into the mouth of a huge and powerful magnet. A reassuring technician Velcro-straps your head down to the slab and places a panic button in your right hand, "Just in case." As the slab slowly rolls in, you feel like you are in a drawer being rolled into the storage cabinet wall of a morgue. The hair on your arms brushes the narrow sides of its walls. Your eyes stare at the seeming-to-move lid a few centimetres from your face. If you do not possess the good sense to close your eyes, which I did not, claustrophobic waves may wash over you, and may begin to drown you, and your thumb may caress the panic button with increasing frequency, and you may push the panic button, and hear the technician's trying-to-calm-you voice as she rolls you out of the magnet, and tells you to "Take some deep breaths" and "Think pleasant thoughts" and "Try closing your eyes next time," before she rolls you back in.

While the magnet rotates around me and my tightly closed eyes, I try to distract claustrophobia's imminent implosion with "pleasant thoughts" of running free in my childhood. The whirling clicks and grinds of the magnet's rotation bring me to a midway ride at the Canadian National Exhibition, called "The Rotor."

My friends and I pilgrimaged to "The Ex" every year on Labour Day weekend, as did tens of thousands of other kids. The guys met at my house early in the morning. We walked the block to catch the bus, then eagerly transferred to a streetcar, then another streetcar, without parental accompaniment since age ten, the year of that first Rotor ride. Our intense anticipation inflated with each clang of the streetcar's overhead cord, pulled by a rider requesting the next stop. We could reach the cord only by standing on a seat, which we only occasionally did, just before we accidentally pulled the cord. Each announcement of the final streets' names bringing us closer to and then through The Ex's massive Dufferin gates was met with exhilarated cheers.

After wildly whooping as we flew off the streetcar, we would run as straight as possible to a roller-coaster–type ride. Unlike my friends, I did not love roller coasters; quite the opposite, the drops terrified me. However, The Rotor terrified my friends, while, for some reason, I found it peaceful. And as I always had to appear courageous to my friends of course, The Rotor became an important part of my childhood.

The Rotor is a round metal room about fifty feet in diameter, covered by a conical tin roof. There are no restraining bars or shoulder harnesses in The Rotor, like those compulsory in the other high-speed rides. Indeed there are no leather straps, or plastic handles, or indeed anything to clutch onto in The Rotor. You just stand against the 360° wall and stare across its vacant diameter at the person standing against the opposite wall.

Soon you hear an ominous metallic thud as the small steel door through which you entered The Rotor, pretending to duck your head while still standing on your tiptoes to meet the height requirement, is shut. Then you hear the scary scrape of rusty steel sliding on rusty steel as the door is bolted shut from the outside. After a second or two of hermetically sealed silence, you hear the molten groan and feel the grating jerk of The Rotor rousing from sleep.

As The Rotor commences a slow rotation, you widen your stance on the corrugated steel floor, bend your knees a bit, spread your arms, and lean harder and harder into the wall behind you. You hear the clacketing of steel wheels increase in frequency and pitch, as they accelerate on what must be a circular steel track below the floor. Soon you no longer have to lean into the wall behind you as your back, then head, then arms have become plastered into it. You cannot move any muscles except your eye muscles. Then, to your shock first time on, the floor drops out, and your eyeballs, which you try hard to restrain from looking down, stupidly stare down into the screaming jaws of the beast below your unsupported feet. You panic, as you are sure that at any second you will slide down the wall to be shredded by its cogs and gears. You mentally try to suction yourself against the wall behind you because you physically can't use the muscles you need to press your back into the wall. As you rotate faster and faster, you stop worrying about sliding down the wall and start worrying that you are going to take off upward like a rocket and crash your head into the metal roof. However, if you are very lucky, you may relax and bask in the peaceful elation of gravity defied.

Too soon The Rotor begins to slow, and you actually do start sliding down the wall, and start clamouring with all your now-working muscles to cling to the wall to avoid being chewed by The Rotor's gears. You slide down anyway, but the floor is miraculously back. You gratefully embrace the solidity of its steel, preferably with your feet, but sometimes with your butt or a shoulder. You hear the bolt outside the door scrape again and the door clang open like on a submarine after surfacing. You follow the curved line of tipsy Rotor riders and wobble along the wall to the door, trying not to bump into the rider ahead or behind you. You wobble through the door to the concrete pavement outside, past a man with a mop and bucket and dangling cigarette to join a chorus of vomitteers, gushing out the corndogs and cotton candy gorged since their arrival at The Ex.

I rode The Rotor many times in the subsequent years of my youth, but always taking a two-hour food pause before ducking through its door, and always wishing the other riders did the same, particularly those who vomited while The Rotor was still in spin. My friends never rode The Rotor again. They roller-coastered while I rotated, personally preferring centrifugal force to gravitational force. When we met at a prescribed time and cotton candy location, they would always shake their heads with a mixture of awe and concern for my sanity when they saw I had once again survived The Rotor intact — that is, with no vomit on my T-shirt. One year The Rotor was no longer there. The midway had become too frivolous for our times anyway.

Lying in the magnet, eyes smiling but firmly shut, brain firmly fixed in my youth, I reach peace, and begin investigating the dichotomy of rotating in The Rotor, centrifugally plastered vertically on its metal wall, and having a magnet rotating around me, gravity and Velcro tape holding me down horizontally to its non-metal slab. I may have fallen asleep, which would not have been unreasonable, considering the MRI began at 2:00 a.m. The next thing I hear is, "It's over" and I feel the drawer being rolled out.

"That wasn't so bad was it," the technician gently soothes, as if I am a child or an elderly person.

I respond, "Next time I want a blindfold like they give you in front of a firing squad."

It is a bad joke, and I am certain I will be punished.

I am called down to see the neurologist the next day. "Normal" would have come over the phone. The MRI showed white specks at the base of my brain and in the brain's balance centre, the cerebellum. These white specks could mean MS. My neurologist remains noncommittal as to their meaning. I am grateful that he thankfully continues to avoid articulating a possible diagnosis.

The episodes of right eyeball's rotating increase in frequency and duration, prompting a second MRI, only three months after my first. The next day, I go over the computer images with one of the neuroradiologists. He stares at the images, lifts his head, and apologizes when he tells me that, "The number of white specks has significantly increased." He looks at my brain's images, then my eyes, back to my brain, and finally settles on my eyes.

"What's going on?" slips from my mouth before I can zip it shut. I can't put it back.

His eyes go back to the MRI images, "I'm sorry, I'm not sure what is going on."

Later in the day, the neurologist echoes, "Not sure."

Two nights later, I bolt upright from sleep with a tremendous headache. I do not get headaches. I am surprised to see a torrent of vomit hurl against the wall on the opposite side of the bedroom. Vomit hits the wall again and again, "projectile vomiting" like Linda Blair's in *The Exorcist*. I have not vomited since my first Rotor ride.

So I know what is going on as I am being driven at full speed to the Emergency Room, vomit bursts slamming the bottom of my bathroom's beige plastic wastebasket. The ER nurses know what is going on as they hurry my stretcher to the MRI suite, after quickly handing me a kidney-shaped aquamarine plastic vomit basin. The MRI technician knows what is going on as she quickly Velcroes down my forehead and rolls me into the magnet, telling me "Try not to vomit." And when she rolls me out of the magnet and I see the Chief of Neurosurgery, the Chief of Neuroradiology, the neurologist-on-call, and my neurologist, wringing eight hands in front of a wall's worth of my brain's computerized images, I definitely know what is going on.

The doctors step toward me in unison, a tight phalanx of sombre centurions. The smile on my face surprises them and makes them feel uncomfortable. The Chief of Neuroradiology casts down his eyes, and reaches out his right hand to my left shoulder.

"Jeff, you've had an event."

When referring to one's brain, "event" is the euphemism for a stroke, usually a thrombotic stroke, as "a bleed" is the euphemism for a hemorrhagic stroke. I test my brain's speech centre with, "Yes, I know." My smile broadens. Their expressions become more grave.

"Do — you — un — der — stand what I mean?" the Chief of Neurology slowly asks, drawing out and emphasizing each syllable.

I laugh, "Yes, I know exactly what you mean."

Then I pump my first "Yes." I test my legs by sliding off the slab and standing. I pump my fist, shout "Yes" again; then raise my arms in Victory's V. I proceed to take a wobbly victory lap around the MRI room, bouncing off the occasional wall. When I return to the doctors, I try to give each a high five. But none of them is interested in high-fiving a once-serious colleague who has clearly been rendered both mentally and physically unbalanced by a stroke.

Their embarrassed eyes surreptitiously flit to one another and then back to the deranged dervish. Most eyes eventually settle on my neurologist. He knows me best. He slowly steps forward, lost in thought. I assume he's contemplating his neuroanatomy knowledge to determine whether the location of my stroke could have, in addition to obviously affecting my brain's balance centre, also affected my brain's mood centre. He puts his right hand on my left shoulder, and says in a very compassionate voice, "Do you understand what we are telling you, Jeff?"

"Yes."

"What do you understand?"

"That I don't have a neurodegenerative disease."

Suddenly I am alone with Ruth. Alone with Ruth in this high-tech room. Ruth is standing, staring at me with a peaceful but quizzical countenance. She wears a peasant dress like they wore in the late sixties and early seventies. A beautiful agate pendant dangles from her neck on a black leather shoelace. Ruth smiles and spreads her arms as she takes in the massive magnet, the myriad of computers with their blue, yellow, green, and red lights. Ruth pirouettes, billowing the base of her dress as she twirls, once, twice, with unseen energy. I watch her dress calm to smoothness as she stops and directs her smile to me.

Ruth seems to be encouraging me. There is no recrimination in her posture. None is necessary, as Ruth knows the guilt I bear, the guilt I feel, from the past. The guilt I will feel in the future when I leave this Hospital and receive all the high-tech care and support I will need. The high-tech care and support that Ruth was denied every time she left this Hospital. The support she was denied that caused her to be admitted that last time and never discharged.

Ruth wants to lift from my shoulders, from my heart, each boulder whose core is filled with concentric layers of guilt. She will assuage my core of guilt by helping me write the story I promised her I would write. The hardest story I will ever write. Because it is about how I let her down in life, in death, and even after, when I struggled to find the courage to put these words on paper. Because it is the story she never had the opportunity to write herself.

Afterword

The years of feeling guilty regarding my lack of intervention and thus complicity in the inadequate access to accommodation and health promotion Ruth received while she lived and how her life ended, were compounded by feeling guilty that I had not yet written the story I promised her I would write. I claimed as placation that I was focused on the best interests of my family, my patients, and my students. I so feared writing this book that I was able to convince myself that I had no time to take it on amidst my clinical, research, teaching, and parenting responsibilities, and that the *Canadian Medical Association Journal* article written in 2001 would suffice. I was able to convince myself that I had no time to write Ruth's story: even though I always seemed to find time for other writing, even though I was becoming increasingly obsessed with how by not writing Ruth's story I continued to let Ruth down after her death as I had let her down during her life. However, when I found myself alone with Ruth in the MRI suite after my stroke, as described in the Epilogue, and was struck by the epiphany that once I was discharged from hospital I would be able to access, indeed would have thrust upon me, all the high-tech support and accommodation that Ruth had been denied, it became impossible for me to defer writing her story any longer. Yet I did defer for several more years.

When I finally allowed myself a zone of solitude within which I could begin imagining the first draft, I found Ruth in the zone with me. Not only because I was writing about her, and as an apology to her, but because of her twenty years of a solitude beyond my imagination, and her deep desire to be permitted to write her way out of her solitude. Ruth just wanted to be able to do what I was now doing, and she could have been able to do what I was now doing if she had only been permitted access to the then readily available technology. Ruth would have poured her heart out through her voice into a microphone attached to her power chair, her words being transferred to text through the software already loaded on her computer. All she needed was a biomedical engineer to do the calibrations so that her chin-operated joystick could be hooked up to her computer. I thought about Ruth as I poured my heart out, too, through my voice into the microphone of my thumb-operated Sanyo microcassette recorder, knowing my words would be transferred to text. But Ruth was not permitted her voice, so she was forced to use mine. While I wrote her story, her voice fuelled my voice; her defiant spirit, keeping her chin up when all around her let her down, constantly full of irrepressible optimism and courage, provided me the courage to write this book.

As I indicated in the Preface, the woman I call Ruth instructed me to use her real name, but I did not because I worried that it would suggest that this book was nonfiction. Although this story is based on true occurrences, I could never assume to know this woman well, let alone convey her lived experience based on the staccato relationship I permitted her. So instead I call this wonderful woman Ruth, because another wonderful woman, Ruth McConnell, my long-time assistant and surrogate mother, was dying of cancer during the early years of writing *Patiently Waiting For* .... I also thought the name Ruth appropriate because of the biblical Ruth, a person at the margins of her society who said, "Whither you will go I will go too," because I believe the Ruth in *Patiently Waiting For* ... not only accompanies me wherever I go but leads me there.

After a while, Catherine Frazee, professor, activist, mentor, was in the zone with us, breathing into me her wisdom and grace. In Chapter 37, I describe the first time

I met Catherine and the inspiration that she provided me and so many others, then and forever. After three years of writing, I emailed Catherine a draft of the manuscript. When Catherine emailed me back telling me how much she liked it, I was as ecstatic as a high-school student whose favourite teacher has just said, "I liked your work," even though Catherine is a decade younger than I. I knew that without Catherine's approval, I could take *Patiently Waiting For ...* no further.

The dates of the chapters are fictional approximations. Unfortunately I have never journalled, even though I encourage my students to journal on a daily basis, and to do so in a deeply reflective manner. Indeed, journalling has become a core curricular endeavour in most health professional programs. I wish we had been aware of and had adopted the practice of journalling when we were medical students. Ruth's story may have been different if we had, not only in the writing, but in the living.

As recounted in Chapter 26, I did call our district's Biomedical Engineering Unit and left a phone message requesting a biomedical engineer to return "Doctor Nisker's" call rather than Jeff Nisker's call in the hope that the "Doctor" prefix would increase the odds of a return call. I did hate playing the "Doctor" card, but, as also described in Chapter 26, I had done so several times before for family members in urgent situations, and recently for a close friend. Ruth, even though I had spoken with her fewer than a dozen times, had become my friend, but not a close friend. Yet the injustice of Ruth having to wait for years to access her computer and the freedom that it would bestow her prompted me without hesitation to ask the biomedical engineer to stay late and see her after hours.

Also as recounted in Chapter 29, the same day that I called our Biomedical Engineering Department, one of the two biomedical engineers did return my call, I did quickly plead

Ruth's situation, immediately making it clear that I was not asking him to see her ahead of someone else, for that would be queue jumping and I teach that queue jumping is unethical in our Health Ethics and Humanities curriculum. Rather, I was asking him to see Ruth after hours, like we health professionals do for family members. I even did say that I would pay him at an overtime rate if he would see her after hours. Fortunately he really did interject before I could embarrass myself further by asking me "Do you not think that every parent of every child with cerebral palsy offers to pay me to see their child after hours?" I had not contemplated that there would be many in our community similarly denied access to accommodative technologies. Of course, I should have.

However the injustice inflicted upon Ruth was not significant enough for me to personally help Ruth overcome the injustice, which I of course could have done by driving her to the United States and paying for a biomedical engineer there to do the calibrations on Ruth's chin and make the computations that would permit the joystick on her chair to operate her computer. When I thought about Ruth, I thought about Ruth as a friend, though I rarely thought about Ruth unless she drove into me in the hallway near my office, or had a nurse call to inform me she had been readmitted to hospital. Although I thought of Ruth as my friend, clearly I never became her friend. I am not sure that rarely thinking about a friend precludes friendship. But I am sure that not being there for a friend does.

Ruth was fond of her neurologist and the Hospital's neurology team, although of course she could never openly display or even admit this to anyone as it would make her appear less hardened, be bad for her reputation, and most important, I believe, make her too open to another disappointment down the road. I also like my neurologist and the neurology team, although, of course, being a doctor and working in the Hospital make my experience far from generalizable to other patients. However, the neurology clinic is never overcrowded, no one seems to wait more than half an hour to be seen, and everyone seems respectful, upbeat, and caring of each other.

This environment is possible in all health clinics if we insist through our votes that we fund adequate numbers of nurses and doctors and units for this to occur, which was the case when I started to practise over thirty years ago, but dissolved in the personal income tax cuts–related health funding cuts of the so-called "fiscally responsible" and definitely socially irresponsible governments. A return to social caring has not occurred because of the self-centredness and greed of those who shield their minds from elementary-school arithmetic to be able to believe personal income taxes can be cut without slashing social services such as health promotion and care.

Instead of blaming the government policies that, by trying to create more "efficiency," created less care and accommodation in delivering health and other social programs, we should blame, as health economist Robert Evans believes, ourselves, referring to Walt Kelly's political comic-strip character Pogo's observation, "We have met the enemy and he is us."

If Ruth read the preceding paragraph, she would say that I was up on my soapbox again, like I am when surrounded by my students. And she would say I should act on what I'm preaching about rather than hoping that informing others will promote social change. I guess this is why I have told you this story. For I believe, as Ruth believed, that story is the most powerful tool we have to effect social change. *Patiently Waiting For ...* is the best way I know to engage the general public who, through their votes, ultimately determine social policy and can change the system that let Ruth down, so that others will be truly accommodated in better health promotion and other social programs. This change can happen only when the prevailing imperatives of our society become equality rather than cost-effectiveness, fairness rather than finance.

I hope the readers of *Patiently Waiting For ...* will find ways to insist on the social changes required to promote equality of access, not only to assistive technologies but to all aspects of accommodation that ultimately would support better health promotion and better healthcare for everyone in their community.

Acknowledgements

As indicated in the Preface, I would first like to thank the woman I refer to as Ruth for what she taught me in the staccato sequences we spent together and for the learning legacy she endowed me. I hope this book fulfills my promise to her. I would also like to again thank Catherine Frazee, activist, author, and recent recipient of the Order of Canada, for her inspiration, for her teachings, and for all that her writings and presentations have provided over the years. I thank Jackie Leach Scully, Professor of Social Ethics & Bioethics at Newcastle University and equal rights activist, for her kind and generous Introduction to this book, and for her many important books. Thank you to director Liza Balkan and actor-singer Sheila Boyd for workshopping a decanted-down play version of *Patiently Waiting For ...* that assisted me in completing this book. I would also like to thank Meredith Levine, journalist and university professor, for her helpful comments on the Epilogue. I thank Susan Cox, sociologist and ethics professor at University of British Columbia, for her suggestions on a very early draft and for our years of research together. I thank Carla Rice, Professor at the University of Guelph and equal rights activist, for her suggestions on a very early draft. I thank Mariko Obokata for her very helpful editorial suggestions and organizational skills. I would also like to thank Kathryn Willms and Caitlin Stewart from Iguana Books for their wonderful assistance. I also thank Katharine Timmins, who has been transcribing my manuscripts for many years, and Jennifer Ryder, research assistant in my health sciences job, who helped me with the research for *Patiently Waiting For ....* Finally I would like to thank Roxanne Mykitiuk, Professor of Law, Osgoode Hall Law School, York University, and Director of its Disability Law Intensive Program. Roxanne, my long-time best friend and so much more, who has taught me through everyday conversations what every clinician, policy maker, indeed citizen should know about "disability," accommodation, and human rights.

Popular References

(in order of appearance)

Music

"Unchained Melody," Alex North (music) and Hy Zaret (lyrics), Righteous Brothers, *Just Once in My Life*, Los Angeles, CA, Philles Records, 1965.

"This Nearly Was Mine," Richard Rodgers (music) and Oscar Hammerstein II (lyrics), Rodgers and Hammerstein, *South Pacific*, New York, Williamson Music, 1949.

"Lady in Red," Chris de Burgh (music and lyrics), Chris de Burgh, *Into the Light*, Hollywood, CA, A&M Records, 1986.

"Billie Jean," Michael Jackson (music and lyrics), Michael Jackson, *Thriller*, New York, Epic, 1982.

Films

Superman, 1978, director Richard Donner

Wizard of Oz, 1939, director Victor Fleming

Saturday Night Fever, 1977, director John Badham

Blood and Sand, 1941, director Rouben Mamoulian

Winning, 1969, director James Goldstone

Joan of Arc, 1948, director Victor Fleming

Patiently Waiting For ...

The Ten Commandments, 1956, director Cecil B. DeMille

The Prime of Miss Jean Brodie, 1969, director Ronald Neame

Horror of Dracula, 1958, director Terence Fisher

Cheech and Chong's *Up in Smoke*, 1978, director, Lou Adler

Rocky, 1976, director John G. Avildsen

Phenomenon, 1996, director Jon Turteltaub

The Elephant Man, 1980, director David Lynch

Alice in Wonderland, 1951, directors Clyde Geronimi, Wilfrid Jackson, and Hamilton Luske

The Goonies, 1985, director Richard Donner

To Kill A Mockingbird, 1962, director Robert Mulligan

Pollyanna, 1960, director David Swift

The Sound of Music, 1965, director Robert Wise

The Great Escape, 1963, director John Sturges

The Bridge on the River Kwai, 1957, director David Lean

Gandhi, 1982, director Richard Attenborough

Casablanca, 1942, director Michael Curtiz

Friendly Persuasion, 1956, director William Wyler

High Noon, 1952, director Fred Zinnemann

My Fair Lady, 1964, director George Cukor

She Done Him Wrong, 1933, director Lowell Sherman

The Miracle Worker, 1962, director Arthur Penn

The Exorcist, 1973, director William Friedkin

Television Programs

Six Million Dollar Man, 1974–1978, program creators: Martin Caidin, Kenneth Johnson

The Twilight Zone, 1959–1964, program creator: Rod Serling; writers: Rod Serling, Alfred Hitchcock, Ray Bradbury *et al.*

Mister Rogers' Neighborhood, 1968–2001, program creator: Fred Rogers

Saturday Night Live, 1974–1985, Billy Crystal's sketches of Fernando Lamas

Star Trek, "The Menagerie," Season 1, Episodes 11 & 12, directed by Marc Daniels (Part I) and Robert Butler (Part II), written by Gene Roddenberry

Chicago Hope, 1994–2000, program creator: David E. Kelley

Books

Alice's Adventures in Wonderland, Lewis Carroll. London: Macmillan, 1865.

The Three Musketeers, Alexandre Dumas, père. London: Hooper, Clark & Co., 1844. (first serialised in the magazine *Le Siècle*)

To Kill a Mockingbird, Harper Lee. Philadelphia: Lippincott, 1960.

Poems

"The Dwarf's Song," Rainer Maria Rilke, *The Selected Poetry of Rainer Maria Rilke*, Stephen Mitchell (transl.). New York: Random House, 1982.

"The Panther," Rainer Maria Rilke, *The Selected Poetry of Rainer Maria Rilke*, Stephen Mitchell (transl.). New York: Random House, 1982.

Video Games

Where in the World Is Carmen Sandiego? 1985, developed Brøderbund Software Inc.

Frogger, 1981, developed by Konami Corp.

Donkey Kong, 1981, creator Shigeru Miyamoto.

Scholarly References

Asch A. and Wasserman D. Making Embryos Healthy or Making Healthy Embryos: How Much of a Difference between Prenatal Treatment and Selection? In Nisker J., Baylis F., Karpin I., McLeod C., and Mykitiuk R. (eds.) *The "Healthy" Embryo: Social, Biomedical, Legal and Philosophical Perspectives.* New York: Cambridge University Press, 2010. pp. 201–19.

Evans R.G. *Getting to the Roots: Health Care Financing and the Inegalitarian Agenda in Canada.* McGill Institute for the Study of Canada Conference, Montreal, PQ. 2002.

Kelly W. *Impollutable Pogo.* New York: Simon and Schuster, 1970.

Lippman A. The Politics of Health: Geneticization v. Health Promotion. In Sherwin S. and Mitchinson W. (eds.) *The Politics of Women's Health: Exploring Agency and Autonomy.* Philadelphia: Temple University Press, 1988. pp. 64–82.

Mykitiuk R. and Penney S. *Screening for "Deficits": The Legal and Ethical Implications of Genetic Screening and Testing to Reduce Health Care Budgets.* Health Law Journal 1995;3:235–68.

Parens E. and Asch A. (eds.) *Prenatal Testing and Disability Rights.* Washington, DC: Georgetown University Press, 2000.

Scully J.L. Drawing Lines, Crossing Lines: Ethics and the Challenge of Disabled Embodiment. *Feminist Theology* 2003;11(3):265–80.

Scully J.L. The Secular Ethics of Liberal Quakerism. In Scully J.L. and Dandelion P. (eds.) *Good and Evil: Quaker Perspectives.* Aldershot: Ashgate, 2007. pp. 219–31.

Scully J.L. *Disability Bioethics: Moral Bodies, Moral Difference.* Lanham: Rowman & Littlefield, 2008.

Scully J.L. Towards a Bioethics of Disability and Impairment. In Atkinson P., Glasner P., and Lock M. (eds.) *Handbook of Genetics and Society: Mapping the New Genomic Era.* London: Routledge, 2009. pp. 367–81.

Scully J.L. and Dandelion P. (eds.) *Good and Evil: Quaker Perspectives.* Aldershot, Hampshire: Ashgate, 2007.

Sherwin S. *No Longer Patient: Feminist Ethics and Health Care.* Philadelphia: Temple University Press, 1992.

Sherwin S. and Mitchinson W. (eds.) *The Politics of Women's Health: Exploring Agency and Autonomy.* Philadelphia: Temple University Press, 1988. pp. 64–82.

Stein J.G. *The Cult of Efficiency.* Toronto: House of Anansi, 2002.

Wasserman D. and Asch A. Understanding the Relationship between Disability and Well-Being. In Bickenbach J.E., Felder F., and Schmitz B. (eds.) *Disability and the Good Human Life.* New York: Cambridge University Press, 2014. pp. 139–67.

Further Readings

To learn more about the challenges faced by persons with disabilities because of the attitudes and inequities in the society in which they live, I suggest the following readings as well as other works of disability scholars and writers such as Jackie Leach Scully (United Kingdom), Adrienne Asch (United States), Catherine Frazee (Canada), Tom Shakespeare (United Kingdom), and Isabel Karpin (Australia). Articles providing information on health policy development and its failure to fund accommodation of disabled persons are also listed below, as are other resources used in the development of this book.

Asch A. and Wasserman D. Making Embryos Healthy or Making Healthy Embryos: How Much of a Difference between Prenatal Treatment and Selection? In Nisker J., Baylis F., Karpin I., McLeod C., and Mykitiuk R. (eds.) *The "Healthy" Embryo: Social, Biomedical, Legal and Philosophical Perspectives.* New York: Cambridge University Press, 2010. pp. 201–19.

Canadian Human Rights Act, RSC 1985, c H-6 (1985).

Cox S.M., Kazubowski-Houston M., and Nisker J. Genetics on Stage: Public Engagement in Health Policy Development on Preimplantation Genetic Diagnosis. *Social Science & Medicine* 2009;68(8):1472–80.

Evans R.G. *Getting to the Roots: Health Care Financing and the Inegalitarian Agenda in Canada.* McGill Institute for the Study of Canada Conference, Montreal, PQ. 2002.

Gibson B.E. and Mykitiuk R. Health care access and support for disabled women in Canada: Falling short of the UN Convention on the Rights of Persons with Disabilities: A Qualitative Study. *Women's Health Issues* 2012;22:e111–18.

Joseph M., Saravanabavan S., and Nisker J. Physicians' Perceptions of Barriers to Equal Access to Reproductive Health Promotion and Care for Women with Mobility Challenges. Forthcoming.

Karpin I. and Savell K. *Perfecting Pregnancy: Law, Disability, and the Future of Reproduction.* New York: Cambridge University Press, 2012.

Lippman A. The Politics of Health: Geneticization v. Health Promotion. In Sherwin S. and Mitchinson W. (eds.) *The Politics of Women's Health: Exploring Agency and Autonomy.* Philadelphia: Temple University Press, 1988. pp. 64–82.

Mykitiuk R. and Nisker J. Social Determinants of "Health" of Embryos. In Nisker J., Baylis F., Karpin I., McLeod C., and Mykitiuk R. (eds.) *The "Healthy" Embryo: Social, Biomedical, Legal and Philosophical Perspectives.* New York: Cambridge University Press, 2010. pp. 116–35.

Mykitiuk R. and Penney S. Screening for "Deficits": The Legal and Ethical Implications of Genetic Screening and Testing to Reduce Health Care Budgets. *Health Law Journal* 1995;3:235–68.

Nisker J. Calcedonies. In Jones T., Wear D., and Friedman L.D. (eds.) *Health Humanities Reader.* New Brunswick, NJ: Rutgers University Press, 2014. pp. 442–76.

Nisker J. Calcedonies: Critical Reflections on Writing Plays to Engage Citizens in Health and Social Policy Development. *Reflective Practice: International and Multidisciplinary Perspectives* 2010;11(4):417–32.

Nisker J. *From Calcedonies to Orchids: Plays Promoting Humanity in Health Policy.* Toronto: Iguana Press, 2012.

Nisker J. The Latest Thorn by Any Other: Germ-line Nuclear Transfer in the Name of "Mitochondrial Replacement." *Journal of Obstetrics and Gynaecology Canada* 2015; 37(9):829–31.

Nisker J. Orchids: Not Necessarily A Gospel. In Murray J. (ed.) *Mappa Mundi: Mapping Culture/Mapping the World.* Windsor: University of Windsor Press, 2001. pp. 61–110.

Nisker J., Baylis F., Karpin I., McLeod C., and Mykitiuk R. (eds.) *The "Healthy" Embryo: Social, Biomedical, Legal and Philosophical Perspectives.* New York: Cambridge University Press, 2010.

Nisker J. and Bergum V. A Child on Her Mind. In Bergum V. and Van Der Zalm J. (eds.) *Mother Life Studies of Mothering Experience.* Edmonton: Pedagon Publishing, 2007. pp. 364–98.

Nisker J., Martin D., Bluhm R., and Daar A. Theatre as a Public Engagement Tool for Health-Policy Development. *Health Policy* 2006;78(2–3):258–71.

Nisker J.A. Chalcedonies. *Canadian Medical Association Journal* 2001;16(1):74–75.

Nisker J.A. Rebuilding Compassionate Canadian Health Care Policy. *Journal of Obstetrics and Gynaecology Canada* 2003;25(1):7–12.

Nisker J.A. and Gore-Langton R.E. Pre-implantation Genetic Diagnosis: A Model of Progress and Concern. *Journal of Obstetrics and Gynaecology Canada* 1995;17(3):247–62.

Ontario Human Rights Code, RSO 1990 c H.19. (1990).

Parens E. and Asch A. (eds.) *Prenatal Testing and Disability Rights.* Washington, DC: Georgetown University Press, 2000.

Rice C., Chandler E., Harrison E., Liddiard K., and Ferrari M. Project Re•Vision: Disability at the Edges of Representation. *Disability & Society* 2015;30(4):513–27.

Scully J.L. *Disability Bioethics: Moral Bodies, Moral Difference.* Lanham: Rowman & Littlefield, 2008.

Scully J.L. Drawing Lines, Crossing Lines: Ethics and the Challenge of Disabled Embodiment. *Feminist Theology* 2003;11(3):265–80.

Scully J.L. The Secular Ethics of Liberal Quakerism. In Scully J.L. and Dandelion P. (eds.) *Good and Evil: Quaker Perspectives.* Aldershot: Ashgate, 2007. pp. 219–31.

Scully J.L. Towards a Bioethics of Disability and Impairment. In Atkinson P., Glasner P., and Lock M. (eds.) *Handbook of Genetics and Society: Mapping the New Genomic Era.* London: Routledge, 2009. pp. 367–81.

Scully J.L. and Dandelion P. (eds.) *Good and Evil: Quaker Perspectives.* Aldershot, Hampshire: Ashgate, 2007.

Shakespeare T. Nasty, Brutish and Short? On the Predicament of Disability and Embodiment. In Bickenbach J.E., Felder F., and Schmitz B. (eds.) *Disability and the Good Human Life.* New York: Cambridge University Press, 2014. pp. 93–112.

Sherwin S. *No Longer Patient: Feminist Ethics and Health Care.* Philadelphia: Temple University Press, 1992.

Sherwin S. and Mitchinson W. (eds.) *The Politics of Women's Health: Exploring Agency and Autonomy.* Philadelphia: Temple University Press, 1988. pp. 64–82.

Stein J.G. *The Cult of Efficiency.* Toronto: House of Anansi, 2002.

United Nations. Convention on the Rights of Persons with Disabilities. Resolution A/61/106 of December 6, 2006. New York: United Nations, 2006.

Vanstone M., King C., de Vrijer B., and Nisker J. Non-invasive Prenatal Testing: Ethics and Policy Considerations. *Journal of Obstetrics and Gynaecology Canada* 2014;36(6):515–26.

Wasserman D. and Asch A. Understanding the Relationship between Disability and Well-Being. In Bickenbach J.E., Felder F., and Schmitz B. (eds.) *Disability and the Good Human Life*. New York: Cambridge University Press, 2014. pp. 139–67.

About the Author

Jeff Nisker MD PhD FRCSC FCAHS

Jeff Nisker is a clinician, researcher, university professor, and writer. His plays and short stories bring the general public, health professionals, and policy makers to the position of persons immersed in the social inequities of new scientific capacities. Jeff has received many research grants in the basic, clinical, and social sciences to study prevention of estrogen-related cancer, ethical and social issues in reproductive genetics, and the lack of accommodation that persons with disabilities receive for health promotion. Jeff has also co-held a Canadian Institutes of Health Research/Health Canada grant to research public engagement and citizen deliberation for health policy development through his innovative use of full-length theatre. Jeff has authored or co-authored over 170 peer-reviewed scientific articles and book chapters, many short stories, and seven plays published in the collection *From Calcedonies to Orchids: Plays Promoting Humanity in Health Policy*. His plays have been performed throughout Canada, in the United States, the United Kingdom, Australia, and South Africa. Jeff has served on the editorial boards of *Journal of Medical Humanities* and *ARS Medica* and is the international representative on the Board of the Centre for Literature and Medicine. Jeff has served national positions such as Co-chair of Health Canada's Advisory Committee on Reproductive and Genetic Technologies; Editor-in-Chief of *Journal of Obstetrics and Gynaecology Canada*; Scientific Officer of the CIHR Peer Review Committee on Health Ethics, Law and Humanities; and Executive of the Canadian Bioethics Society. Jeff has received many research and education awards, including the Society of Obstetricians and Gynaecologists of Canada President's Award for the most significant contribution to the specialty; Western University's Faculty Scholar's Award for Innovation in Research and Education; and, for his plays promoting public engagement in health policy, Canada's Royal Conservatory of Music's Music Excellence in Education Award, which recognizes the efforts of an outstanding educator who embraces the idea that the arts have a capacity to change the world. He was one of the first two obstetrician-gynaecologists inducted into the Canadian Academy of Health Sciences. Through all this, Jeff has maintained his clinical practice in hormone-dependent malignancy, pituitary tumours, and reproductive endocrinology.

Jeff was chosen by the Canadian Broadcasting Corporation's Peter Gzowski as one of the 13 *"Best Minds of Our Time."*

CPSIA information can be obtained at www.ICGtesting.com
Printed in the USA
LVOW07s0533220916

505666LV00001B/5/P